Fourth Edition

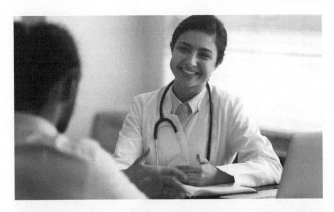

Career Success in Health Care
Professionalism in Action

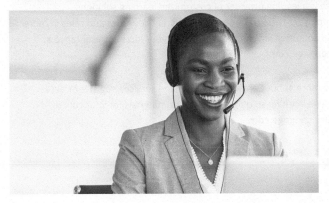
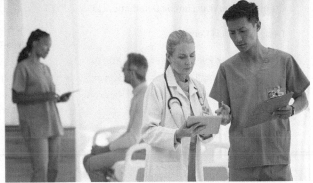

Bruce J. Colbert, MS, RRT

Faculty Emeritus, Associate Professor/Past Allied
Health Director, University of Pittsburgh at
Johnstown, Johnstown, Pennsylvania

Elizabeth D. Katrancha, DNP, CCNS, RN, CNE

Quality Consultant, Accreditation Specialist,
Veteran's Health Administration

✶ Cengage

Australia • Brazil • Canada • Mexico • Singapore • United Kingdom • United States

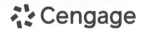

Career Success in Health Care:
Professionalism in Action, **Fourth Edition**
Bruce J. Colbert, MS, RRT;
Elizabeth D. Katrancha, DNP, CCNS, RN, CNE

SVP, Product: Cheryl Costantini

VP, Product: Thais Alencar

Portfolio Product Director: Jason Fremder

Associate Portfolio Product Director: Laura Stewart

Product Manager: Andrea Henderson

Product Assistant: Renee Bunszel

Learning Designer: Deb Myette-Flis

Content Manager: Kate Russillo

Digital Delivery Quality Partner: Lisa Christopher

Director, Product Marketing: Neena Bali

Product Marketing Manager: Joann Gillingham

IP Analyst: Erin McCullough

Production Service: Lumina Datamatics Ltd.

Designer: Felicia Bennett

Cover image(s): PeopleImages.com - Yuri A/Shutterstock.com; fizkes/Shutterstock.com; PeopleImages.com - Yuri A/Shutterstock.com; Rido/Shutterstock.com

For product information and technology assistance, contact us at
Cengage Customer & Sales Support, 1-800-354-9706
or support.cengage.com.

For permission to use material from this text or product, submit all requests online at **www.copyright.com**.

Library of Congress Control Number: 2023951189

ISBN: 978-0-357-93684-9

Cengage
5191 Natorp Boulevard
Mason, OH 45040
USA

Cengage is a leading provider of customized learning solutions with employees residing in nearly 40 different countries and sales in more than 125 countries around the world. Find your local representative at **www.cengage.com**.

To learn more about Cengage platforms and services, register or access your online learning solution, or purchase materials for your course, visit **www.cengage.com**.

Notice to the Reader

Publisher does not warrant or guarantee any of the products described herein or perform any independent analysis in connection with any of the product information contained herein. Publisher does not assume, and expressly disclaims, any obligation to obtain and include information other than that provided to it by the manufacturer. The reader is expressly warned to consider and adopt all safety precautions that might be indicated by the activities described herein and to avoid all potential hazards. By following the instructions contained herein, the reader willingly assumes all risks in connection with such instructions. The publisher makes no representations or warranties of any kind, including but not limited to, the warranties of fitness for particular purpose or merchantability, nor are any such representations implied with respect to the material set forth herein, and the publisher takes no responsibility with respect to such material. The publisher shall not be liable for any special, consequential, or exemplary damages resulting, in whole or part, from the readers' use of, or reliance upon, this material.

Printed at CLDPC, USA, 04-24

This book is dedicated to Pap and Gram Cus;
their love, wisdom, and dedication to education
and family have left a legacy that will last
for generations to come.

Contents

Section 1

Communicating with Yourself: Achieving Personal Excellence

Chapter 1

Study Skills: Laying the Foundation 3

Chapter 2

Characteristics for Personal and Professional Success 27

Chapter 3

Setting Goals and Time Management 55

Chapter 4

Thinking and Reasoning Skills 85

Chapter 5

Stress Management 111

Section 2
Communicating with Others: Achieving Professional Excellence

The major goal of this text is to provide students with an engaging foundation that will ensure success in their chosen health care career and establish them along a pathway as a lifelong learner. This is a lofty but definitely achievable goal.

We all know that health care is one of the fastest growing industries due in part to an aging population and dramatic technological advances. The face of health care is changing rapidly. The changing environment results from a combination of many factors such as pressures for health care reform, a diverse population, and remodeled delivery systems. However, one thing that will never change is the need for highly trained professional health care providers.

About 15 to 20 years ago when our students graduated, employers were asking questions related to their cognitive knowledge (do they know their stuff?) and psychomotor skills (can they perform well?). We rarely, if ever, get those types of questions anymore. Potential employers expect that by virtue of graduation the student has been assessed and proven to have the cognitive and psychomotor skills to function in a chosen profession. The major questions we are now asked about our students are:

Are they good team players?

Do they show up on time?

How are their creative and critical thinking skills?

How well do they handle stressful situations?

Are they good time managers with organizational skills?

Do they accept personal responsibility?

The list goes on, but it is clear that the major concern for employers is the students' behavioral skill sets—this all-encompassing thing we call professionalism. In education, we refer to this as the affective domain and this is usually one of the hardest domains to both assess and teach. Keep in mind that what will set your students apart from other graduates in their career search is how well they perform in the behavioral aspects of their program. Not only is it rewarding when they do well in their career search and land that first position, but the employer's satisfaction and desire to hire more of your program's graduates because of their high level of professionalism sets your program apart.

The authors hope to use their collective wisdom of years of teaching, clinical experience, and offering workshops concerning the affective domain, to produce a text that gives students clear direction and assistance in setting and achieving goals directed toward successful careers in the health professions. In addition, this text will give students both academic and "life" skills that will help them reach their full potential.

Changes to the Fourth Edition

We are gratified that this nontraditional textbook has continued to be successful enough to warrant a fourth edition. Health care schools have come to fully realize the importance of focusing on professionalism and career skills not only for their students' employment success but also for the enhancement of reputation and marketability the school receives from producing students proficient in these areas. In this fourth edition, we have maintained the "easy to read and relate to" writing style that helps to personally connect the material to the individual student's life experience. While easy to read, the text still challenges students to self-assess, think, and apply information for their personal and professional enhancement. The following list represents "What's New" in this fourth edition:

- We have added the integrated assessments and activities within the chapters, as opposed to including them at the end of the chapters, so that students can immediately apply what they are learning.
- We reviewed chapter content, features, art, and activities to ensure the use of inclusive language throughout.
- We updated all figures and photos to make the text visually appealing for all learners.
- We surrounded the worktext with engaging web-based activities, including videos and interactive activities that reinforce the content in a relevant manner.
- We updated MindTap with video-based activities, engagement activities, and assessments throughout in both the cognitive and affective domains.

The following areas of content have been added or enhanced in this fourth edition, specifically with you, the student, in mind:

- Increased self-assessment of current study skills and habits
- Added suggestions for improving study skills such as active reading

- Enhanced evaluation of personal attitudes
- Added SMART system for goal achievement
- Discussed the importance of being organized and added organizational skills development
- Discussed the importance of keeping a schedule
- Enhanced understanding of critical and creative thinking
- Developed activities to integrate critical and creative thinking into everyday life
- Enhanced understanding of stress and developing personalized ways to handle stress
- Expanded on the numerous and varied health care careers
- Enhanced communication skills especially in the area of patient interaction and public speaking
- Expanded on the importance of the health professional's role in patient satisfaction
- Identified the key skills needed for effectively interacting with and meeting the needs of patients and family members in various settings
- Identified ways to find open positions
- Enhanced writing skills for cover letters and resumes
- Identified and expanded upon ethical and legal issues in health care
- Defined and expanded upon infection control
- Expanded coverage of health care to all areas outside of the traditional hospital setting
- Included links to helpful Internet resources for professional organizations, government agencies, and clinically relevant material
- Added appendices of useful health care websites such as infection control, vital sign values, converting measurements, medical terminology, and answers to select feature boxes

Organization of the Text

Career Success in Health Care: Professionalism in Action is organized to maximize the effective development of the softer skills necessary to succeed in the health care professions. The text is overall divided into two sections. Section 1 "Communicating with Yourself: Achieving Personal Excellence" (Chapters 1–5) serves as the foundation to enhance intrapersonal affective skills first before one can effectively communicate with others or develop the interpersonal skills in Section 2.

Chapter 1 lays the foundation with assessments and techniques to maximize study skills. Chapter 2 develops the characteristics needed for personal and professional success. Chapter 3 focuses on setting goals and time management techniques. Chapter 4 develops critical and creative thinking and problem-solving skills. Chapter 5 concludes section one with the development of a personalized stress management system.

Now that Section 1 focused on the individual developing their intrapersonal skills, Section 2 "Communicating with Others: Achieving Professional Excellence" (Chapters 6–11) develops the interpersonal skills needed for health care professionals. Chapter 6 lays the foundation with developing the various types of communication. Chapter 7 deals with communication in action such as customer relations, telephone etiquette, public speaking, and recording and reporting information. Chapter 8 focuses on understanding and maximizing communications within an organization. Chapter 9 develops patient interaction and communication skills. Chapter 10 helps the student in the communications needed to seek out and secure their first career position in health care. Chapter 11 concludes with professionalism in action by developing the issues that will impact the student as they begin their career.

Finally, each chapter is organized in a manner to maximize soft skill development. The student will begin with a self-assessment of the skill being developed, followed by content and exercises meant to enhance that particular skill and then conclude with a personalized action plan to fully develop the skill.

Features of the Text

- The Anticipatory Exercises provide opportunities for students to connect the content to themselves personally through questions that encourage self-reflection.
- The Skill Application activities encourage students to practice skills learned in the chapter and relate those skills to themselves and the workplace.
- With the Test Yourself activities, students complete self-assessments that help them analyze their strengths and identify areas for improvement.
- Just for Fun activities take a lighter approach to the subject material while still teaching the concept.
- Case Studies provide a method to pull several concepts together.
- Internet Activities help further research skills.

Instructor & Student Resources

Additional instructor and student resources for this product are available online. Instructor assets include an Instructor's Manual, Educator's Guide, PowerPoint® slides, Solution and Answer Guide, and a test bank powered by Cognero®. Student assets include PowerPoint® slides. Sign up or sign in at www.cengage.com to search for and access this product and its online resources.

MindTap

MindTap is a fully online, interactive learning experience built upon authoritative Cengage Learning content. By combining readings, multimedia, activities, and assessments into a singular learning path, MindTap elevates learning by providing real-world application to better engage students. Instructors customize the learning path by selecting Cengage Learning resources and adding their own content via apps that integrate into the MindTap framework seamlessly with many learning management systems.

Key features of MindTap include the following:

- Check Your Understanding quizzes measure students' achievement of the most important learning objectives in the chapter.

- The Chapter Quiz provides students opportunities to apply selected chapter concepts based on their personal experiences.

- The Apply It: Video Quiz provides students with authentic, application-based video assignments for practice in applying chapter concepts in a real-world context.

- The Chapter Test assesses students' achievement of selected learning objectives in the chapter; some learning objectives require a specific assignment to measure achievement.

To learn more, visit www.cengage.com/training/mindtap.

We truly hope this project and the enhancements made to the fourth edition assist health care students in fully realizing their potential, not just in their chosen career but also in life.

Developing Portfolios

The difference between ordinary and extraordinary is that little extra.

—Author Unknown

During a focus group discussion conducted by the National Center on Education, business personnel were asked about assessment and hiring practices. Many agreed with one person who stated, "When I'm considering applicants for a job, I want them to be able to show me some examples of schoolwork and what they can do … the trouble is, I don't see many students who can present themselves like that."

Of course, this quote will *not* pertain to you. You will be able to showcase your talents and land that job or that seat in the school of your choice. Developing an active portfolio within MindTap will ensure your success. Although portfolios may be somewhat new to classrooms, for years artists, actors, models, journalists, writers, and academicians have been successfully using this concept.

What is a portfolio, and what can it do for you? First, there are many answers to what a portfolio is and what kinds of things should go into its development. One definition states that a portfolio is a systematic and continuous process that continually changes as the learner grows and develops their literary and personal skills. This definition seems very technical and not very personal.

Simply stated, a portfolio is a collection of the learner's *work* that can demonstrate their progress. For example, an artist's portfolio may contain representative samples of the artist's art. These art samples will be selected to show the artist's talents, styles, and growth. As you work through this project, you will learn things that will help you develop skills and gain knowledge that can be presented in your portfolio. The portfolio will become a powerful and friendly tool to help you develop personally and professionally.

The main goal of an effective portfolio is to promote active learners who can assess and examine their growth over time. Additional goals that the portfolio will accomplish include:

- Helping students and teachers develop and evaluate meaningful goals
- Assisting students in self-assessment skills
- Creating action plans for development and improvement
- Developing a sense of process and organizational skills
- Enhancing written and oral communication skills
- Emphasizing student responsibility in teaching and learning
- Linking curriculum instruction and assessment to the school and community

Teachers, parents, peers, or school administrators can have input into your portfolio. However, you should organize it and make sure it is showing how you are developing and improving. For example, your text will help you develop long-range career and educational goals. These would be good to include in your portfolio. These goals may change over time and need updating, but they will give you a focus or direction as to where you are going. The text and accompanying MindTap will also help you to develop a powerful résumé that will serve as a keystone of your portfolio.

Acknowledgments

We wish to acknowledge all the quality health career teachers we have met through our interactive lectures and workshops. You truly are a fun and motivated group. In addition, we wish to thank all those at Cengage who made this innovative project possible. Especially noteworthy are **Andrea Henderson**, **Deb Myette-Flis**, and **Kate Russillo** who not only believed in the project and helped shaped the outcome, but were so nice to work with.

The authors also wish to acknowledge all the instructors who reviewed the manuscripts of each edition and provided valuable comments that continue to help this project evolve. The reviewers include:

Reviewers of the Fourth Edition

Alexandra K. Fiore (Kennedy), B.P.S. Online Faculty Administrator
Bryant & Stratton College
Buffalo, NY

Timothy Demchak, Ph.D., LAT, ATC Professor
Indiana State University College of Health and Human Services
Terre Haute, Indiana

Marilyn Martin, B.S.B.A., M.B.A. Instructor
Central Piedmont Community College
Charlotte, North Carolina

Dr. Denise Pruitt Program Chair and Professor
Mass Bay Community College
Wesley, Massachusetts

Reviewers of the Third Edition

Christie Taylor, RN, BSN, MSEd Health Occupations Instructor
Tyrone Area High School
Tyrone, Pennsylvania

Dorothy Winger, MS, CFCS Health Occupations and Family/
	Consumer Sciences Teacher
Wisconsin Health Occupations Professional Educators (HOPE) and
	Wisconsin Association of Family and Consumer Sciences (WAFCS)
Madison, Wisconsin

Reviewers of the Second Edition

Gwen Barnett, BS, MT (ASCP) Health Science Education Instructor
North High School
Evansville, Indiana

Mary Beth Brown, MRC, BA Annually Contract Faculty
Sinclair Community College
Dayton, Ohio

Roxann DeLaet, RN, MS Professor
Sinclair Community College
Dayton, Ohio

Vicki Gentzel, BS Health Careers Recruitment/Retention Specialist
Harrisburg Area Community College
Harrisburg, Pennsylvania

Tina M. Peer, BSN, RN Instructor
Registered Nursing and Allied Health Programs
College of Southern Idaho
Twin Falls, Idaho

Maggie Thomas, PT, MA PTA Program Coordinator
Kirkwood Community College
Cedar Rapids, Iowa

Robert W. Wilcosky, MEd, RRT Professor Emeritus/Advisor
Medical Center Campus
Miami Dade College
Miami, Florida

About the Authors

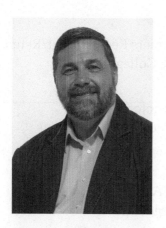

Bruce Colbert is a clinical associate professor and past director of the Allied Health Department at the University of Pittsburgh at Johnstown. He has authored 14 books and has given over 300 invited lectures and workshops at both the regional and national level. Many of his workshops are devoted to how to teach professionalism; improving active teaching skills, stress and time management; enhancing critical and creative thinking; and developing effective decision-making skills. He is an avid basketball player who is awkwardly trying to now transition to golf.

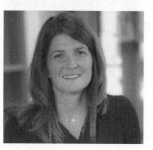

Elizabeth Katrancha is a quality consultant, accreditation specialist for the veteran's health administration. She has a background as a professor of nursing. She is acutely aware of the soft skills that are needed in the next generation of health care professionals. She has published numerous clinical articles.

Message to the Student

If we are headed in the wrong direction and do nothing to alter our course, chances are we will end up there.

— **Old Chinese Proverb**

This text is not about math or science. It will not ask you to memorize massive amounts of information or complex formulas. This book is about *you*. What do you wish to become, and how do you plan on getting there?

This text explores who you are. This should be a hard but worthwhile exploration. Your education can be the ticket to this wondrous and productive journey, but only you can choose the path and determine how hard you are going to work. Sounds corny and you may have heard it all before, but think about it.

Right now you are preparing for the rest of your life. The knowledge and skills you obtain within this text along with your clinical skills and showcasing yourself in a positive manner can help you achieve your full potential. Section 1 of the text focuses on self-communication. This section focuses on *you*. Only you can ensure that you achieve personal and professional excellence. Therefore, the most important personal relationship you must first establish is with yourself.

We all know how crucial good communication skills can be in our relationships with others. But what about communication within ourselves? Positive self-communication is the "foundation" upon which to build a successful personal and professional life.

Section 1 will help you determine your strengths and identify areas for improvement of your *intra*personal skills (intra = within). It will assist you in developing action plans and achievable goals to improve your chance of success. It will make you think about who you are and what you wish to become.

Section 2 looks at and improves your communication skills with others, or your *inter*personal skills (inter = between). This section discusses communication at an interpersonal level within a group, team, or organization. Basic communication skills are stressed along with their application to success within your first career position.

In addition, Section 2 focuses on job-seeking skills. It emphasizes that the time to prepare for gainful employment is *right now!* This is why branding and showcasing yourself and self-assessment are common themes throughout this text. You will analyze and build upon strengths. You will also identify areas that need improvement with a corresponding action plan.

This will not be a passive journey, and you will be expected to be an active participant in this process. This text has integrated exercises designed to complement and reinforce the topics under discussion. You will be instructed to *stop* and complete those exercises to further develop the concept. This integrated text will then assist you in developing ways that will showcase who you are and what you can do.

Please keep in mind that all learning does not take place in the classroom and you are fortunate in health care that you get to "try on" your profession in the clinical setting. Always put your best foot forward no matter whether in the classroom, lab, or clinical setting. In clinicals especially, take time to learn about the whole team and not just your assigned patients. Finally, understand that your behavioral tone in your program will directly relate to your future career success.

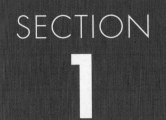

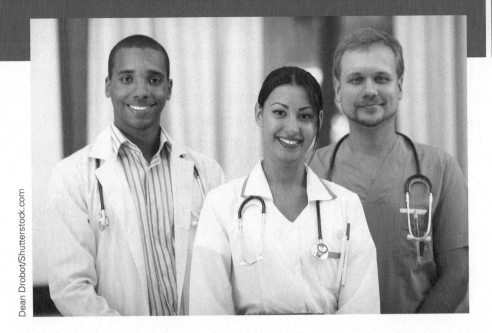

Dean Drobot/Shutterstock.com

Communicating with Yourself: Achieving Personal Excellence

This section focuses on *you!* Only you can ensure that you achieve personal and professional excellence. The first and most important relationship you must establish is with yourself. Positive self-communication is the "foundation" upon which to build a successful personal and professional life. The following chapters will be covered in this section:

In this section, you will get to know who you are and how you think. You will assess your intrapersonal skills in areas such as study skills, professional attitude, goal setting, time management, stress management, critical thinking, and decision-making skills. You will then develop action plans specific to you and your life to fully realize your personal and professional excellence in your chosen health care career.

Chapter 1

Study Skills: Laying the Foundation

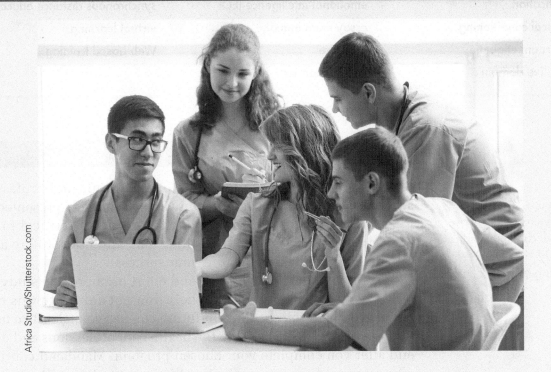

Africa Studio/Shutterstock.com

Objectives

Upon completion of this chapter, you should be able to:

1. Relate the importance of good study habits to your personal success.

2. Perform an assessment of your current study skills.

3. Formulate a plan for improvement of study skills.

4. Based on the learning process, develop strategies to improve test-taking skills.

5. Relate the importance of health and good study skills.

6. Identify success strategies for online courses.

7. Develop strategies for "branding" or "showcasing" yourself as a successful student and a future employee.

Key Terms

acronym	continuing education credits	mnemonics
active reader	critical thinking	objective examination
affective domain	distance learning/education	passive reader
asynchronous distance education	e-learning	psychomotor domain
certification	emotional intelligence (EQ)	synchronous distance education
classical conditioning	essay examination	virtual learning
classroom etiquette	licensure	Web-based training
cognitive domain	lifelong learner	

Introduction

The principal goal of education is to create men and women . . . who have minds which can be critical, can verify, and not accept everything they are offered.

—Jean Piaget

Study skills are essential for both your academic and professional success. This is the reason the study skills section is presented first. Even though this is a relatively small chapter, it is critical for your success. Therefore, spend the initial time and effort to lay a solid foundation upon which to build your success.

An initial investment of time and effort in improving study skills will pay off in a big way. It will help you not only with this course but also with all the current and future courses you take. The need to be a **lifelong learner** is vital in the health care professions and doesn't end after you complete your chosen program. Mandated **continuing education credits** and **certification/licensure** testing will require you to maintain your study skills throughout your professional career. This chapter discusses five important ingredients that help make studying successful. For all chapters, personalized activities will follow discussion to immediately reinforce these concepts.

Anticipatory Exercise 1–1   Why Should You Commit?

Before we begin discussing specific techniques, it is important for you to *believe* in the importance of enhancing your personal study skills and how it will enhance your personal and professional lives. Make a list of five specific things good study skill habits can do for you *now* and in the *future*.

_____

_____

_____

_____

_____

Daily Study Preparation

There is *no* substitute for daily preparation. On the surface, it may seem as if this will take a lot of time, but if done correctly, it will actually save a tremendous amount of time. Daily preparation includes developing a schedule plan that budgets your time. This allows you to use the whole day, do things in proper order, reduce the confusion in your life, and have a better sense of accomplishment.

Do not be discouraged if your first few schedules do not work well. Build in some flexibility. Do not forget to schedule relaxation and recreational time as these are also important. Studies show you learn more in three 30-minute sessions than in one 2-hour session. Therefore, studying notes over shorter periods in more frequent intervals is more effective than long cramming sessions. Use 1 hour as your *maximum* study time without a break.

Another useful technique is to take advantage of "wasted" time. For example, you might take your medical terminology note cards with you to your physician's visit. You can now study them while you are waiting and won't even be upset if your appointment is late because you can use the valuable time to study for your upcoming exam. Commuting students can record formulas, definitions, and other needed study concepts and listen to them during their commute to school or clinical practicum. Smartphones have many useful "apps" such as medical terminologies, review questions, and educational games that can also serve to reinforce study concepts during these so-called wasted time periods.

Organizing your study space and materials is also a critical preparation step. Keep in mind that there is no one magical way to organize, and certain ideas may work better for you. However, it is important to keep your organizational system simple and consistent whether you use a tablet, smartphone, or large desk calendar as your organizational tool.

For example, keeping a color-coded notebook for each class will assist your daily preparation and organization. Some students find it more convenient to use three-ring binders and three-hole-punch handouts, exams, assignments, and so on, to maintain all materials in one organized binder.

Laptops and tablets are being used more within the classroom. If you are using one, make sure you keep your electronic notes and files organized as well in labeled and dated folders. Make sure you backup all your information on a regular schedule. Also, be careful to avoid the nonstudy-related distractions a laptop or tablet may tempt you with while either taking class notes or studying for an exam.

Skill Application 1-1 Developing Your Study Schedule

Attempt to make a weekly schedule that sets aside time for study. Allow each study block a maximum of 1 hour. Do not forget to add your recreational activities. It may take several schedules before you get all the bugs out. Also, this is just a guide; you must always have flexibility for unexpected events. Figure 1–1 shows a sample schedule.

The key is to set aside enough study time to properly prepare and stick to a schedule that works for you. Even if you have all your work done, do not skip a study block. Instead, review your notes or "quiz" yourself.

Remember, only you can determine the schedule that is right for your life. Using Figure 1–2, make your own study schedule. Photocopy the blank schedule so you have several extras or create the grid electronically. Now attempt to follow this schedule and modify it accordingly until you develop a schedule that works for you. You are encouraged to work with teachers, family members, and friends to help develop and modify the schedule. Post your final schedule in your *special* study place.

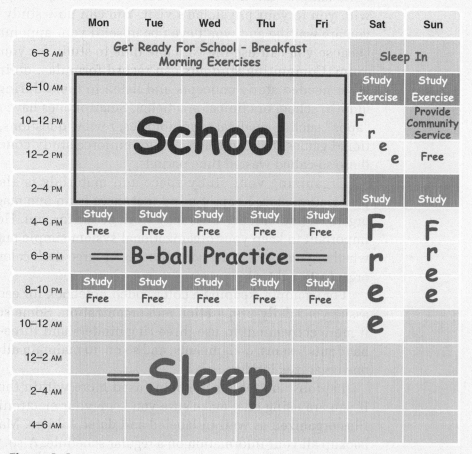

Figure 1–1
Sample study schedule.

(continues)

(continued)

	Mon	Tue	Wed	Thu	Fri	Sat	Sun
6–8 AM							
8–10 AM							
10–12 PM							
12–2 PM							
2–4 PM							
4–6 PM							
6–8 PM							
8–10 PM							
10–12 AM							
12–2 AM							
2–4 AM							
4–6 AM							

Figure 1–2
Fill in your study schedule (you may want to make some blank copies first).

Select a Good Time and Place of Study

The time you choose to study is very important. It may not be the same time for all of us. Some people are "morning people," whereas others are not. We all have different biological clocks, so try to schedule times when you are most alert and focused.

The place you choose to study is also important. Ideally, it should be the same place each time, so that you "connect" this place to studying and consequently become focused. It should have minimal or no distractions and good lighting. The table or desk should have only the tools of study, not distractions or mementos that may lead to daydreaming.

Have you ever heard of **classical conditioning**? The term came from an experiment performed on dogs. In this experiment, a bell was rung and dogs were then fed meat. The meat caused the dogs to salivate.

Again and again, experimenters would ring a bell and feed the dogs. After much repetition, the dogs connected the ringing of the bell to the meat. A bell only had to be rung for the dogs to salivate, even if they were not given meat. What is the purpose of telling you this story other than making you hungry or grossing you out?

When you study in bed and then go to sleep repeatedly, you soon connect studying to sleeping (Figure 1–3). Every time you begin to study in bed (even in midafternoon), you may begin to yawn and not be as focused. You are conditioning yourself to connect studying to sleeping. Simply avoid studying before sleeping because you will not be as focused and, therefore, will be less effective. Besides, studying in bed may interfere with your ability to get a good night's sleep.

Figure 1–3
Is this the best way to study?

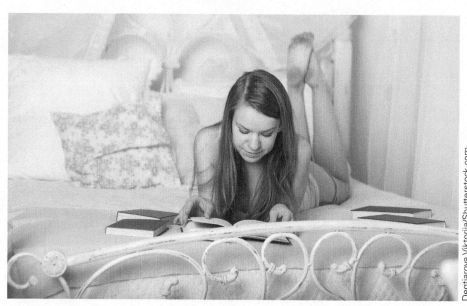

Degtiarova Viktoriia/Shutterstock.com

Test Yourself 1–1

Finding the Right Time and Place

Assess your current place of study by answering the following questions. Be critical and honestly circle the response that best answers the question.

1. Do you study in the same place each time?	Mostly	Sometimes	Rarely
2. Is it quiet where you study?	Mostly	Sometimes	Rarely
3. Are the conditions and lighting comfortable?	Mostly	Sometimes	Rarely
4. Do you have all the tools (e.g., pencils, rulers, computer, paper) you need to study at this place?	Mostly	Sometimes	Rarely
5. Do you limit distractions such as cell phones during study time?	Mostly	Sometimes	Rarely

Skill Application 1–2 **Developing Your Personalized Action Plan**

How well did you do on Test Yourself 1–1? It does not matter as long as you were honest. Remember this is an assessment of where you are now. Your eventual goal should be to have all your responses be "Mostly." If they are now, great! If not, you need to develop an action plan to make all the responses "Mostly" in the near future.

For each question that did not have a "Mostly" response, develop an action plan that states specifically what you need to do to make the response "Mostly" in the future. Include a statement about when it will be accomplished. A sample action plan is shown in Figure 1–4. Now complete your action plans.

Figure 1–4
A sample action plan.

Date of plan: 10-10-24

Goal: To improve my study environment

Plan: I will improve the lighting in my room by adding a desk lamp. In addition, I will clean my study desk and organize my work area.

Date accomplished: 10-20-24

Evaluation: This has improved the study area. However, I need to get a higher-watt lightbulb to see better.

Finally, classical conditioning can also be used to your advantage in health care, especially during your clinical experiences. Repeated positive interactions and therapies with a patient will "classically condition" the patient to feel good each time they see you.

Use Good Study Habits

The study habits we will explore include note-taking, active reading, and classroom behavior or **classroom etiquette**. All three areas need to be fully developed to truly realize your full academic potential.

Note-Taking

Take good, accurate, legible notes. Remember that the purpose of taking notes is to get key points from textbooks and lectures, not to write every word that is said or written. Listen much and write a little.

It is important to be prepared to take notes when class begins by having your notebook, pen, laptop, and any handouts or readings at hand. Try to participate actively and constructively in class discussions and do not hesitate to ask questions. Pay attention not only to what the teacher is saying but also to how they say it. For example, if the teacher says "to summarize" or "the main points are," then this material should be written down along with anything that is written on the board or screen.

Instead of highlighting the chapter, outline your chapters so that you can make the connection from your brain to the pencil. This is what you will need to do when taking the test. Outlining may initially take longer than highlighting, but you will learn the material better. Outlining actually saves studying time in the long run. Review your lecture and outline notes frequently.

Also make diagrams and pictures to help visualize concepts within your outline. The more you can "see it," the better you can understand relationships or how it all fits together. As an example, see Figure 1–5 for a visual representation of how you might visualize the concepts covered in this chapter leading to your success.

Figure 1–5
Visualize the steps to your success.

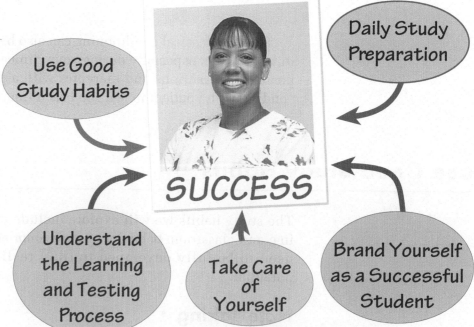

Skill Application 1–3 Developing Good Study Habits

Take a sample chapter from an assigned reading and outline the material. Remember to focus on key points. An outline of this chapter on study skills is provided as an example.

Sample Outline

Study Skills
Introduction
The need to be a lifelong learner is vital due to continuing education, certification, and licensure mandates.

A. Daily study preparation.

   1. Make up study schedule that works for me.

   2. Keep study sessions to 30–60 minutes.

B. Select good time and place to study.

   1. *Do not* study in bed.

   2. Choose place with minimal distractions.

   3. Have good lighting.

   4. Make sure table or desk has only needed study tools.

   5. Limit distractions.

C. Use good study habits.

   1. Take good notes (accurate and legible).

   2. Outline chapters instead of highlighting.

   3. Utilize active reading principles.

   4. Periodically review notes.

   5. Teach aloud to others.

   6. Practice good classroom etiquette.

D. Understand the learning and testing process.

   1. Educational domains.

      a. Cognitive domain—domain associated with learning facts and theories.

      b. Psychomotor domain—domain of learning skills.

      c. Affective domain—domain associated with developing professional attitudes and behaviors, emotional intelligence, or soft skills.

(continues)

(continued)

> **E.** Critical thinking and memory.
>
> **1.** Try to "truly learn the material" and use memorization only as an aid.
>
> **2.** Use acronyms (words made from first letter of other words).
>
> **3.** Use other memory aids (mnemonics) such as rhymes or stories.
>
> **4.** Test-taking skills.
>
> **5.** Be prepared for different types of examinations and review old tests.
>
> **F.** Take care of yourself.
>
> **1.** Eat right, exercise, and stay drug free.
>
> **2.** Get plenty of rest, especially before an examination.
>
> **G.** Study skills for online courses.
>
> **1.** Most programs have some form of online learning.
>
> **2.** Online courses require self-discipline and self-motivation.
>
> **3.** Use the assessments and strategies in this chapter to succeed.
>
> **H.** Branding yourself as a successful student.
>
> **1.** How do you want your teachers to see you?
>
> **2.** Show willingness to work hard and develop positive academic relationships.
>
> **3.** Be dependable and on time for class and with assignments.
>
> **4.** Take responsibility for your actions and always strive to improve.

Did outlining the chapter help to create an organized overview? _____

Did you understand the material better by physically outlining the chapter? _____

List three reading assignments you can outline in the coming week. _____

_____

_____

_____

_____

Active Reading

Do you consider yourself an **active** or **passive reader**? If you simply read the material but do not comprehend much of what you have just read or lose your focus, you are a passive reader. This inefficient reading method wastes your valuable time and impacts your academic performance. Active readers want to understand and remember what was just read. They increase their comprehension by writing notes as they read, asking themselves questions about what they are reading, and even marking their text with notes. While this takes more time and effort initially, you will need less time to review for the exam and be better prepared to get a good grade.

A simple way to remain in the active reading mode is to periodically ask yourself questions about what you have just read. If you cannot answer these questions, you probably are losing interest and need to take a short break, clear your head, and become more focused.

Another active reading strategy is to preview the assignment by skimming chapter headings, subheadings, bolded terms, figures, and chapter summaries, to get a feel for the chapter first before you read every word. Outlining and taking notes while reading is a very effective active reading technique.

Active reading can also be facilitated by marking your text or handouts with notes. Many students may hesitate to mark their textbook because they might want to resell it. However, studies show that students who mark their textbook while they read learn the material better. You can write notes in the margins or on figures to help visualize and relate the material. Figure 1–6 shows an example of a marked-up figure to help active reading and studying.

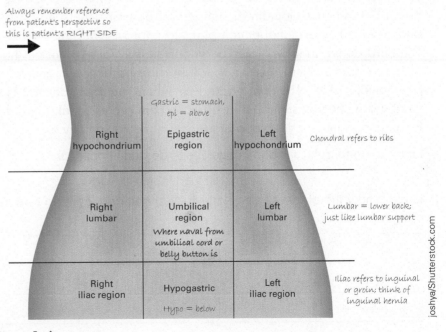

Figure 1–6
Anatomy and physiology marked up figure example to enhance active reading and help in studying and understanding the material.

You can even make your studying more active. Study with a friend and explain concepts to each other. Each time you explain something, the oral recitation reinforces your understanding. You will soon learn that "there is no better way to learn something than to teach it out loud to someone else."

Classroom Etiquette

Simply put: Be responsible and go to class! Attending class and being on time shows your instructor respect and that you value your education. This will carry over into your clinical experience and showcase your professionalism. Read the assigned readings before class. This will also help you begin to develop professional responsibility skills that are critical in health care. Consider sitting near the front so that you are less tempted to be distracted by side conversations, both personal and electronic. Get in the habit of turning off your phone before entering a classroom just like you would a concert or public event so that you can fully focus on the lecture.

Food for Thought 1–1

Ancient Wisdom

There are three educational domains or areas you need to concentrate your studies on. The most familiar to you is probably the cognitive or knowledge domain. For example, studying and learning your medical terminology so you can pass the exam is the cognitive domain. This book is mainly about the affective domain or behavioral domain where you are performing self-assessments and developing personal action plans to improve your interpersonal and professional skill set. The third domain that will also be important for your success in health care is the psychomotor or performance skills domain. Your laboratory practice in clinical skill areas will improve your psychomotor skills. The total package is when you are proficient in all these domains and this is what will make you stand out as a health care professional. Read this ancient quote and relate it to the importance of your laboratory and clinical experiences.

I hear and I forget. I see and I remember. I do and I understand.

—Confucius

Explain how the above quote relates to studying and learning and the educational domains.

_____

_____

_____

_____

Understand the Learning and Testing Process

There is a lot more to the learning process than meets the eye. For example, did you know there are three distinct educational domains and each has its own unique assessment, learning, and teaching styles?

Educational Domains

You may ask, "What does this have to do with me—isn't this something for the teacher?" The answer is yes, this is very important for the teacher; however, if you understand the concepts, it will greatly help you to understand the learning process and how to succeed within your program and beyond.

The three educational domains are the **cognitive, psychomotor,** and **affective domains.** We will begin with the cognitive domain since this should be the one you are most familiar with.

Cognitive Domain. The cognitive domain comprises assessing, teaching, and learning theories and facts. This domain establishes your knowledge and your ability to apply it to your chosen area of study. You have been immersed in this domain from the beginning of your educational process through sitting in lectures, reading texts, and taking examinations. Psychologist Benjamin Bloom studied this domain extensively, and it is important to understand his "take-home" messages.

He found that it is essential to learning that you begin with a foundation of knowledge and build on it in a systematic manner. He developed a taxonomy (classification system) of the increasing levels of the six cognitive areas: knowledge, comprehension, application, analysis, synthesis, and evaluation.

He showed that to truly learn you must begin with the foundation (knowledge) and learn definitions and recognize information before you can move on to higher levels such as application and synthesis. This is why you begin with learning all those medical word roots and abbreviations in medical terminology and not complicated case studies that require evaluation.

So whether you are teaching or learning, you must begin with a solid foundation of knowledge (be able to list and define medical terms) before you can apply what you learned to a new situation or evaluate a case study full of medical terminologies. Cognitive assessment can be done with objective testing that includes multiple-choice, short answer, essay, and case study questions. In essence cognitive testing is all about finding out if you "know your stuff."

Psychomotor Domain. Having chosen the health care profession, you will be expected to perform well in this education domain that focuses on your skills. For example, performing cardiopulmonary resuscitation or CPR is a psychomotor skill that requires you to perform this vital procedure. You certainly must have the higher cognitive knowledge to know "when to perform CPR," but now you must actually learn and *do* the skill.

The psychomotor skill development requires guidance and demonstration (usually in lab) followed by repetition until the skill is done successfully. The cognitive domain should be integrated while doing the psychomotor skill. For example, if you are performing a blood pressure test in lab, you should be able not only to perform the skill but also to answer cognitive questions, such as what are normal readings or how do you adapt to take an infant's blood pressure. This forces you to have to think while doing the skill, so it becomes second nature.

Affective Domain. This domain focuses on assessing and developing professional attitudes and behaviors. Increasingly, this domain is becoming more emphasized as employers focus on hiring individuals who excel in this domain. In the past, employers asked about your cognitive knowledge and skills but now they expect you have them upon graduation and are more interested in your professional attitude. Will you show up on time? Are you a good team player? How well do you get along with others? Do you have leadership qualities?

These skills are sometimes referred to as the "soft skills" and even special terms such as your **emotional intelligence (EQ)**. However you term it, it all boils down to developing a professional attitude coupled with a high level of interpersonal skills that include your ability to handle stress, manage your time, communicate effectively, make informed decisions, work on a team, demonstrate leadership, and so on. These soft skills are difficult to teach and often hard to learn or more precisely internalize as a set of values and beliefs. This is what this interactive text is all about. Your cognitive skills will develop in the classroom and your psychomotor skills will be developed in your labs and with repetition and practice. However, your affective skills are what will set you apart and especially become critical when you enter your clinical practice or practicum experience.

This textbook is not set up like your medical terminology book because you do not teach and learn in the affective domain the same way you do for the cognitive domain. This is one reason why it is more difficult to teach and learn in the affective domain. The guiding principles for the affective domain and indeed the writing and development of this textbook are as follows:

1. The three A's of affective teaching/learning must be adhered to in order. First is *Assessment* to see where you are currently with a skill. This is establishing a baseline. The next "A" is *Awareness* where you become aware of techniques, methods, and so on to improve this affective skill, whatever it is. The final "A" is developing an *Action Plan* based on your assessment and awareness to enhance the chosen affective skill.

2. Affective domain concepts are shorter and less cognitive in nature. In other words, it has just enough cognitive theory to make

the behavioral concept relevant. It should, therefore, motivate you to engage in the affective skill and not get lost in the cognitive theory. You should understand WHY this particular behavioral skill is important for your success and HOW you can improve it.

3. Like Bloom's cognitive taxonomy that began with a solid knowledge foundation before moving on to higher level cognitive skills, you must establish a solid affective foundation in areas such as stress and time management before you can become proficient with higher level behavioral skills. Simply put, how can you make good decisions or interact well with others, if you are always stressed out or do not manage your time well? This is why the textbook builds on the affective skills and also focuses on "yourself" in Section 1 before moving on to skills that require high levels of interactions in Section 2.

Critical Thinking and Memory

To succeed, it is important to truly "learn" the material and use **critical thinking** skills to assist in problem solving. *Critical thinking* has many definitions, but most emphasize the ability to gather and analyze information in order to solve problems or create new opportunities. Critical thinking is goal-oriented and focuses on a purpose.

One who can think critically knows how to obtain information, understand it, and apply it. This is a step above merely memorizing information for short-term storage.

Say, for example, you memorize the steps to CPR. However, you do not truly understand *why* you need to establish an open airway, or even *how* to actually do it. You may be able to repeat the steps on a pen and paper test and receive a good grade. However, what if in 6 months you are in a situation in which you need to perform CPR on an individual in need? You cannot say, "I had that 6 months ago and I really didn't learn the material."

Education is to encourage thinking skills rather than memorization, but you have to recognize that memory is vital. Memory is used as an index of success because most techniques used to measure learning rely on it. Therefore, a good memory is definitely an asset that you should develop.

Try to memorize only when you are well rested. Also use memorization techniques such as the use of **mnemonics**. Mnemonics are words, rhymes, or formulas that aid your memory. **Acronyms** are one type of mnemonic. An acronym is a word made from the first letters of other words. For example, *HOMES* can help you list the five great lakes (Huron, Ontario, Michigan, Erie, and Superior). The ABCs of CPR remind you that *A* = establish **A**irway, *B* = rescue **B**reathing, and *C* = establish **C**irculation. This helps you better remember the steps and their proper order in a critical situation. Figure 1–7 illustrates an acronym and a picture to aid in learning the steps to take during a hospital fire.

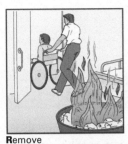
Remove

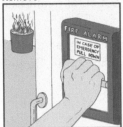
Activate

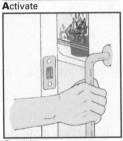
Contain

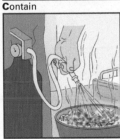
Extinguish or

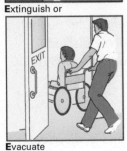
Evacuate

Figure 1–7
An acronym (RACE) and visual representation aid in learning the steps to take during a hospital fire.

You can also use rhymes or formulas to assist memory. For example, "spring forward, fall back" helps us remember to adjust our clocks accordingly when daylight savings time was in use. You can also make up silly stories to help remember facts. In fact, often the sillier the story, the easier it is to remember.

Skill Application 1–4 Helping Memory Skills

This chapter stresses the importance of learning versus memorization. However, it discusses that a good memory is an essential ingredient to the learning process. Let us do some mental gymnastics to build your memory capabilities.

An acronym is a word that comes from the first letters of other words. For example, the treatment for a sprain is to **R**est, put **I**ce on it, **C**ompress the affected area, and **E**levate the sprain. To help you remember this treatment, you can form the following acronym:

R: Rest

I: Ice

C: Compression

E: Elevate

This could easily help you remember this for a test or when you have to put it into use in a tense situation.

As health care shifts its focus toward prevention, you may see the treatment of a sprain to include "Prevention" techniques such as stretching and warm-ups. How could you easily incorporate this into a revised acronym?

_____

See if you can come up with an acronym for the following:

1. The types of cuts are punctures, incisions, lacerations, and abrasions.

   Acronym: _____

2. A nursing progress note consists of four main parts: A *subjective* response from the patient, *objective* patient information, *assessment* of patient, and a *plan* of action. We discuss what each of these areas means in depth later. For now, see if you can come up with an easy way to remember subjective, objective, assessment, and plan.

   Acronym: _____

3. The nursing progress notes can also be expanded to include *intervention* and *evaluation*. What could these notes be now called?

   Acronym: _____

Answers can be found in Appendix F.

Just For

FUN 1-1

Acronyms and Mnemonics

Not all acronyms spell a perfect word. For example, the four main types of tissues within the body are epithelial, muscular, nervous, and connective tissues. One acronym is C-MEN. You may also need to add vowels to form recognizable terms.

You can also use mnemonics such as rhymes or formulas to help your memory. For example, "My Very Educated Mother Just Served Us Nachos" tells you the planets within our solar system in order from the sun. You may not know which M is for Mercury and which is for Mars, but use your intuition. Mercury is in a thermometer and relates to heat and, therefore, is closer (hotter) to the sun. Your memory combined with your thinking skills can be very powerful.

Try to make up a mnemonic for the following:

1. Lines of a treble clef: E, G, B, D, F
Mnemonic: _____

2. Colors in the spectrum: red, orange, yellow, green, blue, indigo, and violet
Mnemonic: _____

3. The body's vital signs: pulse, respirations, temperature, and blood pressure
Mnemonic: _____

Answers can be found in Appendix F, but you could come up with something different as long as it makes sense to you and aids your memory skill.

Test-Taking

When taking examinations, the best advice is to be prepared. If you have prepared daily, you should have no problem. Studying for the test should be reviewing what you already know.

Know what type of test you are taking. With an **objective examination** (multiple choice, true/false), be sure you understand all directions first. With objective examinations, usually your first idea about the answer is your best. One strategy is to cover the answers with a piece of paper and then think of the answer in your head. Then uncover the answer and select which option was closest to what was in your head. Again, some strategies will work better for you than others so select the ones that best fit you. Be careful with multiple choice to pay attention to qualifiers such as all, most, none, never, and so on.

If it is a subjective **essay examination** (short answer), survey the questions, plan your time, and give time to questions in proportion to their value. Title your essay as this will focus your thoughts. It is sometimes valuable to sketch out or outline your response so it will be better organized. Look at clues in the questions, such as "compare and contrast" means to first write similarities and then contrast the differences. Other key essay terms and meanings:

Define: Provide definition and explanation of concept

Discuss: Consider possible points of view on the concept

Argue: Present an opinion in an informed manner

Apply: Show use for

Make sure you proofread your answers for errors and spelling, and if written out, make sure your handwriting is neat and easy to read. If the teacher has to work or strain to read it, it will most likely impact your grades.

Some people develop their own test-taking strategies. They may do all the easy questions first and then return to the more difficult ones. Make sure you mark the questions you skipped or you may forget to return to them. Finally, do not destroy your old examinations—keep them and learn from them!

Take Care of Yourself

Learning requires a healthy mind, body, and attitude. It is important to exercise your brain to stay mentally fit, but it is also important to stay physically fit. Eating right, exercising several times a week, and not abusing drugs or alcohol will make you feel better and enhance your ability to learn. There may be times you must study when sick, tired, or fatigued. Begin these study sessions with slow rhythmic breathing. This helps you relax and in turn improves concentration. Remember to get sufficient rest, especially before examinations.

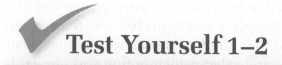 **Test Yourself 1–2**

Do You Take Care of Yourself?

A future chapter discusses the importance of proper exercise, nutrition, and healthy living habits. In that chapter, you will make a thorough assessment and develop an action plan for a healthier you. For now, circle the answer to the following general questions and make an action plan for each "yes" answer(s).

(continues)

(continued)

1. Do you feel tired during the day when you are studying? Yes No
2. Do you take any mood-altering drugs? Remember alcohol and cigarettes are included in this category. Yes No
3. Do you forget to exercise during the week? Yes No
4. Do you eat a diet that is heavy in fats and "junk food"? Yes No

For each of your "Yes" answers develop a specific action plan.

Your action plan:
Date of plan: _____
Goal: _____
Specific plan: _____
Date accomplished: _____
Evaluation: _____

Your action plan:
Date of plan: _____
Goal: _____
Specific plan: _____
Date accomplished: _____
Evaluation: _____

Remember to implement and evaluate your plans!

Study Success Skills for Online Courses

While much of health care education is provided in the classroom, in clinical simulation laboratory, and during your clinical practicums, it is likely you will have some online education as part of your coursework. Online education is technically any learning that occurs through the Internet and includes terms such as **distance learning/ education**, **virtual learning**, **e-learning**, and **Web-based training**. Many of these platforms such as webinars will become more prominent for continuing education once within your profession. As online learning continues to grow and evolve, it becomes important to have both an understanding of online education and specific strategies for success (Figure 1–8).

A huge misperception concerning distance learning is that online courses are easier. In fact, these courses can be more difficult for some students because they require substantial self-discipline and

Figure 1–8
Online education is
becoming more prevalent.

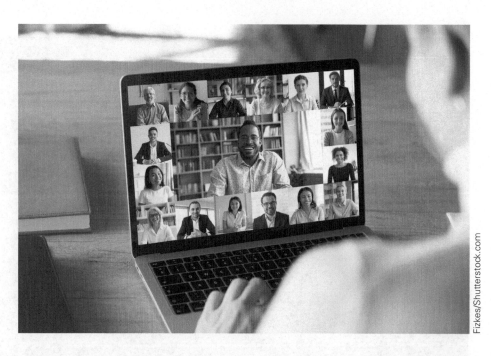

Fizkes/Shutterstock.com

self-motivation. Students who are self-motivated when they begin studying online, can find these types of courses to be rewarding. Do the assessment at the end of this section to determine your compatibility for online learning.

Another misconception is that all online courses are the same. In fact, there are several types of online course formats and experiences. Currently, online courses are broken down into **synchronous** and **asynchronous distance education**. Synchronous courses could include Skype or similar video chat software where students have face-to-face contact with faculty on a regular basis. In essence, you are logged on at the same time as your faculty and fellow students. Asynchronous courses use online bulletin board postings, chat rooms, and text dialogues to conduct the course. In these courses, you may never really see the professor (other than maybe a video introduction) but interact through messaging and postings. Some courses are hybrids and have some face-to-face interaction integrated with text dialogue and postings. In most courses, students sign in at least once a week for a live chat format and conversation to a common board that everyone can read. In addition, weekly assignments and session questions are posted in a "course room" or assignment outline. Tests are usually given in a secure online location where students can access the test or an assigned project or paper.

Here are some specific strategies that will help ensure your success with distance learning:

- Stay self-motivated and read postings daily from your classmates and professor.
- Stay connected and respond via posts on a regular basis to show your unique contribution to the discussion.

- Practice good time management by balancing your personal obligations and meeting all your deadlines.
- Maintain an ideal study environment with all your needed technology and no distractions (remember to avoid the distractions your devices may tempt you with!).
- Use proper APA or MLA citation when writing or posting.
- Participate in any online training or orientation sessions.
- Keep a backup copy of all work e-mailed to your instructor.

Test Yourself 1–3

How Compatible Are Your Study and Academic Habits to Distance Learning?

Answer the following questions either yes or no.

_____ I'm a self-motivated individual.

_____ I rarely procrastinate on assignments.

_____ I have good keyboard, computer, and reading comprehension skills.

_____ I complete all my assignments on time.

_____ I have Internet access and all the technology and software needed for an online course.

Answering "yes" to all these questions will help you to be successful online. If you do have a "no" answer, come up with a specific action plan to change it to a "yes."

Action plan

_____

_____

_____

Branding Yourself as a Successful Student

You may have heard the term *branding* in reference to developing yourself as a recognizable brand to make you stand out. While this is an often-used term, the authors of this text prefer the word *showcasing*. To some, branding may imply slick marketing schemes and we prefer a term with more authenticity. In other words, it means putting your best authentic self in the forefront for others to see. How do you want the world to see you? What can you do to showcase yourself in a positive way? This chapter dealt with academic issues and you should now have the tools to showcase yourself as a great student. We finish this chapter with our top five items that should pertain to you as you present yourself academically within your chosen program:

1. Willingness to work hard, get good grades, and actively participate in all aspects (classroom, lab, clinical) of your educational program.

2. Developing positive relationships with faculty, fellow students, and others at your school or clinical site.

3. Demonstrating a dependable reputation by being on time for class and assignments, working well with others, and doing your fair share.

4. Showing a positive attitude toward learning and having your education as a priority in your life.

5. Taking responsibility for your behavior and always striving for improvement (Figure 1–9).

Figure 1–9
Always keep your ultimate goals in mind!

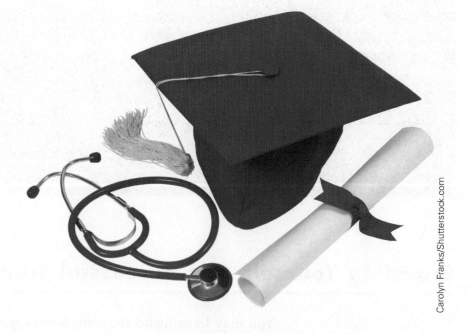

Carolyn Franks/Shutterstock.com

Summary

- The need to embrace being a lifelong learner is vital in health care due to mandated continuing education, certification, and licensure requirements.
- Study skills are a critical element of your current and future success. The five key ingredients to effective study skills are daily study preparation and planning, choosing the proper time and place, using good study habits, understanding the learning process, and taking care of yourself. Taking care of your physical self is crucial for your optimal mental functioning.
- Skills this chapter will help you assess and enhance are organization, note-taking, active reading, proper classroom etiquette, test-taking, and memory skills.

These skills can be applied to any learning environment and will assist you in your career as you become a lifelong learner.
- You must also become a proficient learner in all three educational domains to become a successful health care professional. In other words, you must know your stuff (cognitive domain), be able to perform the skills (psychomotor domain), and demonstrate professional behaviors (affective domain).
- In addition, this chapter discussed personal assessments and skills and strategies to become a successful online learner.
- Finally, the importance of branding or showcasing yourself as a successful student must begin on day one, and several strategies were explored.

Case Study 1–1

Karla was an excellent student in high school, who in her own words "hardly ever took a book home or studied." However, she is now in a health care program, which is much faster paced and more demanding than high school. She can't seem to keep up with all the extra readings and is doing poorly on her exams.

What do you think is the main reason for Karla performing poorly?

_____

_____

What would you suggest she do to turn this situation around in a positive direction?

_____

_____

Internet Activities

Using Internet search engines, try to find additional material on studying that can help you and your fellow students. Some suggested keywords are study skills, active reading, memory aids, and test-taking. Write down something new that you found and can share.

_____

_____

For your chosen health care profession, respond to the following:

Identify any entry-level examinations required for employment.

_____

_____

List the required licensure and certifications.

_____

_____

List any continuing education units (CEUs) requirements.

_____

_____

Congratulations on your work concerning study skills. The time you invested will pay great dividends in your life. Use these skills in this and other courses, and they will serve you well.

Know Where to Get Help

Your school will have study support services such as learning skill centers, peer tutors, math centers, writing assistance, and so on. List the school information here for easy reference.

Resource Center Name: _____

Location: _____

Phone number: _____

E-mail address: _____

Chapter 2

Characteristics for Personal and Professional Success

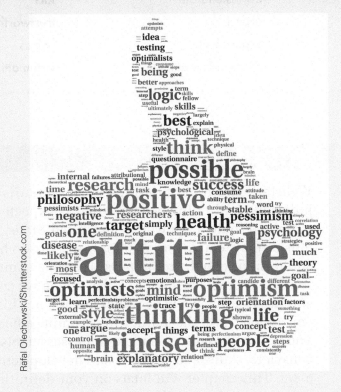

Rafal Olechowski/Shutterstock.com

Objectives

Upon completion of this chapter, you should be able to:

1. Define "success" in your own terms.

2. Relate concepts of values, self-esteem, and a self-confident attitude toward *your* life.

3. Assess your level of assertiveness.

4. Identify ways to improve your personal and professional attitudes.

5. Incorporate a positive and professional image in dealing with others.

6. Identify your own personal "brand".

Key Terms

advocating	honesty	self-esteem
assertive	negative attitude	self-motivation
brand	positive attitude	service industry
caring attitude	profession	sincerity
competency	professionalism	tact
dependability	respect	trustworthy attitude
empathy	responsibility	values
evidence-based practice	self-confident attitude	victim attitude

Introduction

You don't become a good sailor by sailing calm seas.

—John Maxwell

Webster's dictionary defines **professionalism** as the skill, good judgment, and polite behavior that is expected from a person who is trained to do a job well. The United States Department of Labor tells us that "employers want new workers to be responsible, ethical and team oriented, and to possess strong communication, interpersonal, and problem solving skills." When we combine this definition and these skills, we have professionalism. This text will help guide you as you travel the journey to becoming a health care professional. You will be asked to complete self-assessments and to evaluate your behaviors, skills, and attitudes and develop action plans for improvement. This chapter will focus on your definition of success and the attitudes necessary to be successful in today's fast-paced health care environment. You will make mistakes throughout your life; everyone does. It is important that you learn from your mistakes, adjust, and do not keep repeating the same mistakes. A true professional attempts to learn something from each interaction that occurs.

You can get lost in all the *self* terms. For example, people talk about self-esteem, self-concept, self-responsibility, self-management, self-awareness, self-help, and so on. It is easy to get confused by all those terms. Where do you start so that you are not overwhelmed?

We think the answer is **self-motivation**. Self-motivation is one of the characteristics that most influences a person's behavior. In other words, do you want something badly enough to put in the work to achieve your goals? That is something that cannot be taught but must come from within. However, having that motivation or internal drive is not enough. You must combine motivation with an awareness of yourself and develop certain skills to realize your full potential. If you have the internal drive, this chapter gives you the awareness. The remaining chapters in this section build on this awareness and give you the life skills to achieve your goals.

Anticipatory Exercise 2–1   **What Is Success?**

The following is attributed to the American writer Ralph Waldo Emerson.

Success

To laugh often and much; to win the respect of intelligent people and the affection of children; to earn the appreciation of honest critics and endure the betrayal of false friends; to appreciate beauty; to find the best in others; to leave the world a bit better, whether by a healthy child, a garden patch or a redeemed social condition; to know even one life has breathed easier because you have lived.

This is to have succeeded.

What do you think about Mr. Emerson's definition? Write a paragraph about what has the most meaning to you in his writing.

_____

_____

_____

Although we stated you cannot teach self-motivation, you can foster an environment where it will develop. The first step is to look at how you feel about yourself and work on your internal environment.

Everyone has a different definition of what success is. It is important for you to have a clear definition of what you believe is success. It can have many parts to it. Some parts can be short-term and accomplished within a few months or a year, while others may take several years to achieve. For example, hopefully one short-term goal is the successful completion of your health care courses for this year. A long-term goal may be the securing of a professional job in your chosen area. While this is *your* definition, please exercise one caution. Too often in our society, success is equated to money or accumulation of material possessions. Although this may be part of your success goals, try not to make it your sole focus. Look within, for no matter how much your net worth is, it does not mean very much if you are not happy with yourself or your situation.

Self-Esteem

What is **self-esteem**? Simply stated, it is how *you* feel about yourself. Other words for self-esteem are *self-belief* or *self-concept*. Regardless of the term used, this is probably one of the most important questions you need to answer in your life. The way you feel about yourself affects every aspect of your life. In fact, many studies show that there is a direct relationship between self-esteem and academic performance. Simply put, the better you feel about yourself, the better you will do in school. The better you do in school, the better your chance for a successful and fulfilling life. In addition, having good self-esteem enhances your ability to interact with others in a positive way. This is a prime ingredient for any health care provider.

Self-esteem is shaped by your **values**. Values are what you believe in. They are your own thoughts and feelings about yourself. They are composed of the following:

1. What you think
2. How you feel
3. How you act based on how you think and feel

For example, you may *value* competency in an individual. **Competency** means someone is capable of doing something well. Therefore, you "think" as a future health care professional that you should be competent. Emotionally, you "feel" good when you are competent at a procedure and uncomfortable when you are not. Finally, you "act" on these feelings. You may practice a procedure more and more until you become comfortable with it.

How did your values come about? They formed as you developed. Your values were (and are still being) influenced by family, friends, teachers, and the society in which you live.

Attitudes arise from values. For example, you value the concept of honesty. Therefore, you should be honest in your words and deeds. Because you value honesty, you will not lie in your relationships with others. You will be viewed as someone who can be trusted and be truthful in any situation. Figure 2–1 shows how positive values can be shaped.

Figure 2–1
How positive values are shaped.

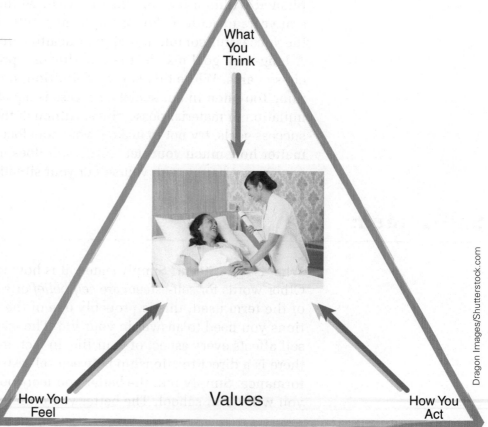

What You Think

How You Feel   Values   How You Act

Dragon Images/Shutterstock.com

Skill Application 2–1 **Your Own Definition of Success**

1. List three people you know personally, whom you consider to be successful.

    a. _____

    b. _____

    c. _____

2. What is it about these individuals that led you to call them successful? Write a short paragraph for each individual to answer this question.

    _____

    _____

    _____

    _____

3. Who are your heroes? Why are they your heroes? Pick one and write all the reasons why you admire this person.

    _____

    _____

    _____

    _____

4. In one paragraph, state your definition of success.

    _____

    _____

    _____

5. List five characteristics you have that will help you become successful.

    a. _____

    b. _____

    c. _____

    d. _____

    e. _____

6. List two short-term success goals (accomplished within 1 year).

    a. _____

    b. _____

7. List two long-term success goals (accomplished within 5 years).

    a. _____

    b. _____

Note: We will talk more about how to write goals in Chapter 3. For now, just write your goal in your own words.

Self-Confident Attitude

A **self-confident attitude** is important for health care professionals (and actually everyone). Being self-confident means you know yourself inside and out. You have assessed your strengths and weaknesses and are confident in what you can do. You believe in your ability to do things and make things happen in a positive manner. Patients react positively to a self-confident attitude; even if you are nervous, you need to put on a "professional face" that is the product of preparation and self-confidence. This does not mean you should overstep your skills or abilities, part of this is having the self-confidence to admit when you do not know something.

Another component of a self-confident attitude is the ability to be **assertive**. An appropriately assertive and self-confident attitude is important in health care. You are responsible for **advocating** for your patient's well-being. Advocating means that you are often the "voice of the patient." For example, what if a physician prescribes a medication dosage that you are sure is incorrect? Do you give the dosage because the physician prescribed it? Or do you call and double-check, even though you may get yelled at for questioning the physician's orders? What would you do in this situation?

Here is one final word to the wise. Anything can be taken to an extreme. Assertiveness taken to the extreme becomes aggressiveness. Self-confidence taken to the extreme becomes obnoxiousness.

Test Yourself 2–1

How Assertive Are You?

1. I can express my feelings easily.	Mostly	Sometimes	Rarely
2. I tell a person when I do not like what they said or did.	Mostly	Sometimes	Rarely
3. I tell people what to do directly.	Mostly	Sometimes	Rarely
4. I do not allow people to take advantage of me.	Mostly	Sometimes	Rarely
5. I am not afraid to tell others the truth about how I feel.	Mostly	Sometimes	Rarely
6. I see the necessity of expressing my feelings to someone else.	Mostly	Sometimes	Rarely
7. I can say "no" to people without feeling bad.	Mostly	Sometimes	Rarely

If you are an assertive person, you should have majority *Mostly* answers with no *Rarely* answers. If you do have *Rarely* answers, this is an area that needs improvement. But how do you improve? Let us say you answered *Rarely* to number 7. You fear telling someone "no" because you think they might not like you. How can you overcome this? One way is through role-playing. You can practice with a friend. Remember, to get good at something takes practice. Have your friend assume the role of someone who is asking a favor of you. Imagine that your friend is asking you to work Friday night. However, you have an important date and say no. As in real life, have your friend really not hear you say no and continue to try to persuade you and make you feel guilty, to get a yes response. Practice saying no and not feeling bad with your friend. By practicing in this made-up scenario, you will be better prepared next time it happens to you in real life.

Food **for** Thought 2–1

Do You Walk the Walk or Talk the Talk?

Have you ever heard someone say another person has an "attitude"? This can be good or bad depending on how the person says it or what that person's attitude is when they say it. An *attitude* is a state of mind. It is how you feel about a person, object, or situation. Your attitudes can be picked up by others. An attitude can be shown by your outward physical appearance or expressions (body language). Attitudes can come through when you talk and interact with others.

Have you ever heard someone say that another person "walks the walk"? This means the person truly lives their values. In this case, personal attitude is consistent with personal values. The person acts the way they believe.

But what if someone just "talks the talk"? This means what the person states is their values are not consistent with their words or deeds. For example, as a health professional, you will be asked to educate your patients on health promotion. Let's say that it is your job to stress the importance of taking care of yourself and taking your medications on time and in a responsible manner. However, you come into the room 10 minutes late smelling of cigarette smoke. Would what you say really be effective? How would you feel if this happened to you?

Skill Application 2–2 **Taking a Look at Yourself**

What are your values? How do they shape your attitudes? These are important questions. You may not be happy with all that you find. Congratulations. This means you are working hard and being honest. We all have some values that should be questioned and attitudes that need work. The first step is to assess our values and attitudes and then to improve upon them.

Complete the following sentences.

1. I am good at _____.

2. The three most important things in my life are _____.

3. I want people to remember me as someone who _____.

4. The most important thing someone can do with their life is _____.

5. I like people who _____.

6. I get angry when _____.

7. The most important attitude in a relationship is _____.

The answers to these questions can begin to tell you a little about your attitude.

Skill Application 2–3 Your Values

We discussed in this chapter how a value arises from the following:

1. What you think

2. How you feel

3. How you act on those feelings

For each of the values, state how you think, feel, and act in your own words. An example is done for you.

Open-minded: *I "think" open-mindedness is important in dealing with people and situations. I "feel" upset when someone is not open-minded about my opinion. I will "act" to become more open-minded when others disagree or have a different viewpoint.*

Kind: _____

_____

_____

Accepting/Inclusive: _____

_____

Cheerful: _____

_____

Competent: _____

_____

Courteous: _____

_____

Forgiving: _____

_____

Helpful: _____

_____

Honest: _____

_____

Empathetic: _____

_____

Responsible: _____

_____

(continues)

(continued)

Your Attitudes

1. List and describe five values or characteristics that you think are important for a self-motivated attitude.

   a. _____

   b. _____

   c. _____

   d. _____

   e. _____

2. You never get a second chance to make a first impression. What attitude would make a good first impression on you?

   _____

   _____

What Is a Professional Attitude?

You have chosen the health occupations. This is a **service industry**, which means you are providing a service to others. In this case, the others are in great need because their health is vitally important. This is also a **profession**, which means it sets high standards for those who claim to be professional. Therefore, it is important for you to develop the personal and professional attitudes that will make you stand out as a competent health care professional.

Remember a time when you or someone you know interacted with a health care professional? Were they professional? What is a professional attitude? The listing of the traits or characteristics of a health care professional can be extensive. However, they can be grouped into three categories as to what most people expect from a professional health care provider. People expect to be treated by a *trustworthy*, *caring*, and *competent* individual. These characteristics and attitudes should become part of your personality.

Trustworthy Attitude

Patients, coworkers, and supervisors must trust you. Patients are literally placing their most precious possession, their lives, in your hands. Many things that are said during their stay could be highly confidential. They must be able to depend on you in their time of need.

A **trustworthy attitude**, Figure 2–2, consists of three main ingredients:

* Honesty
* Dependability
* Responsibility

Honesty means to be truthful. This will help establish trust in a patient relationship. **Dependability** means people can count on you to be there. They can depend on your arriving on time for their treatment. This includes being on time for school and work. Your attendance record is an important reflection on your motivation. Responsibility is fulfilling your obligation to do something. It also means you are accountable and take **responsibility** for what you have done and how well you have done it. It means when you are taught a new skill or ability, you have taken the time to understand and ask questions before applying the skill to the care of a patient.

Figure 2–2
The ingredients of a trustworthy attitude.

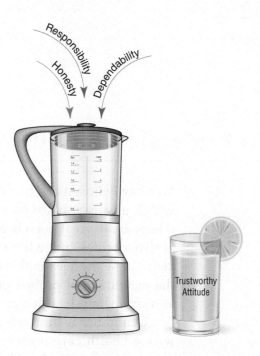

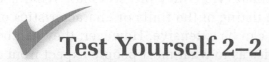

Test Yourself 2–2

Trustworthy Attitude

1. I am honest with others.	Always	Sometimes	Rarely
2. I get to work/school on time.	Always	Sometimes	Rarely
3. I take pride in my work.	Always	Sometimes	Rarely
4. I own up to my mistakes.	Always	Sometimes	Rarely
5. I keep my promises.	Always	Sometimes	Rarely

Caring Attitude

Have you heard of TLC? It stands for tender loving care. To some, it may sound wimpy, but consider this. You are in a strange environment (hospital), and you have just been told you have a critical medical problem that requires immediate treatment. The chances are 50/50 you will survive. You are frightened and you have several questions. No matter who you are, a caring and concerned health care professional would certainly be welcomed at this time.

A **caring attitude**, Figure 2–3, comprises the following:

- Sincerity and empathy
- Respect
- Tact

Figure 2–3
The ingredients of a caring attitude.

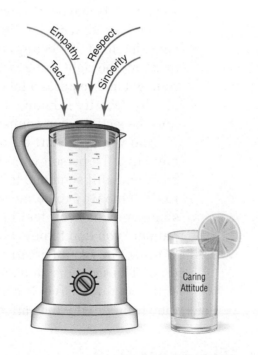

Food **for** Thought 2–2

Being Tactful

Tact is rubbing out another's mistake instead of rubbing it in.

—Author Unknown

Give an example of when you applied this quote (were tactful) in your life.

_____

_____

Sincerity means you *genuinely* care about another individual. Patients are highly perceptive and can spot a phony quickly. They are usually so focused on their caregiver that they can pick up on someone "acting" like they care. A measure of one's sincerity is their ability to empathize with patients. **Empathy** is the ability to identify with and understand another person's feelings, situation, and motives. It means you can understand and are compassionate toward what another person is going through. It also means not being judgmental.

Respect means you treat others with consideration. It means you are kind and courteous about the patient's needs. You do not burst in while a patient is taking a bath or having an uncomfortable procedure done. You respect the patient's privacy and territory. Always remember it is the patient's room, and you are the guest. Say please and thank you. Treat people with patience and tolerance. Calmly react to any given patient or situation. It means that despite what your personal beliefs maybe, you will respect the patient and their choices.

Tact is a term often used in dealing with patients. Tact means being considerate of the feelings of others in difficult situations. It is saying or doing the right thing. This is a difficult skill in the hospital environment and requires a lot of practice. An example of tact is related to obesity. Obesity is known to cause many health issues. However, you must be tactful when counseling a patient about their weight.

Many people start off on the wrong foot by using a "you" statement to tell a person what they should think, feel, or do. Would you be offended if someone told you how to feel, what to think, or what to do? One way to be more tactful is to use an "I" statement to tell someone what you feel or need. For example, instead of telling a patient "*you* don't know how to take your medication correctly," say "*I* think you would greatly benefit from taking your medication like this." The second statement does not put down or blame the patient and is not offensive. It can also be helpful to ask the patient what they want or why they are refusing something.

✔ Test Yourself 2–3

Caring Attitude

1. I get along with others.	Mostly	Sometimes	Rarely
2. I treat everyone equally.	Mostly	Sometimes	Rarely
3. I am polite and courteous.	Mostly	Sometimes	Rarely
4. I can make people feel comfortable in uncomfortable situations.	Mostly	Sometimes	Rarely
5. I can "feel" for someone else or their situation.	Mostly	Sometimes	Rarely
6. I respect other's privacy.	Mostly	Sometimes	Rarely

Again, *Mostly* responses should be your goal.

Competent Attitude

You certainly want someone who is treating you for an illness or accident to know what they are doing. You must have a competent attitude so that your patients will have faith in your abilities to bring them through a crisis.

Competency means that you can perform a certain task. You are proficient. Proficiency means you can accurately, and in a timely manner, follow the approved steps and procedures to get the job done well. A competent attitude, Figure 2–4, consists of the following ingredients:

- Willingness to learn
- Willingness to change
- Acceptance of criticism
- Enthusiasm for learning

To be competent in the health care profession, you must be self-motivated and have a desire and willingness to learn.

You must be willing to learn on a continual basis. New techniques and equipment are constantly being developed. You need to keep up to date and be willing to continue your education to maintain your competency.

Closely related to this is a willingness to change. Health care changes because of research findings, new inventions and technologies, and many other factors. People tend to resist change. However, new research findings in health care may state a drug is not as effective as once thought because of a mutated virus. We must change our treatment according to the current evidence for the good of our patients.

Figure 2–4
The ingredients of a competent attitude.

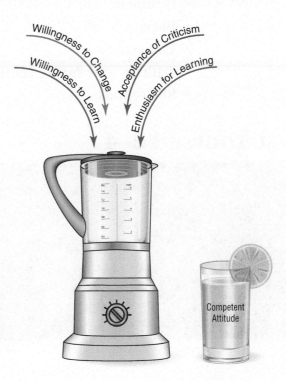

Evidence-based practice utilizes valid well-studied treatment results to direct practice and not just what you "feel" is best for the patient.

A competent person also listens to others' evaluations of their interaction with patients or their performance of techniques. We must, therefore, accept constructive criticism. We learn from our mistakes and the mistakes of others if we have the proper attitude. Constructive (proper) criticism from coworkers, teachers, friends, or patients can help us become better at what we do. After all, this is what we are striving for.

Remember that mistakes are not failures. We all make mistakes and can use them to improve our future performance. When you make a mistake as a health care professional, a specific procedure is followed. Let us say you made a drug medication error. An *incident report* would be filled out by you and your supervisor. The goal is not to punish but to evaluate why it happened and to *prevent* future errors. This can lead to overall improvements for workers and patients alike. Honesty plays a large role in this situation; you must be honest and admit mistakes so that the root cause can be identified, and future errors prevented.

Everyone gets criticism. Unfortunately, it is not always done properly or constructively. We will discuss how to give constructive criticism to others in upcoming chapters. For now, however, there are certain behaviors that are unprofessional when being criticized. The following is a list of negative reactions to criticisms. You should *NOT* do the following:

- Get angry
- Make excuses
- Complain
- Blame others
- Whine or cry
- Criticize your supervisor in turn
- Run or walk away

Test Yourself 2–4

Competent Attitude

1.	I continually strive to improve.	Mostly	Sometimes	Rarely
2.	I accept criticism easily.	Mostly	Sometimes	Rarely
3.	I enjoy learning new skills.	Mostly	Sometimes	Rarely
4.	I work with enthusiasm.	Mostly	Sometimes	Rarely
5.	I can accept change.	Mostly	Sometimes	Rarely

A Look at Idioms

Different societies have different combinations of words or expressions that are particular to them. These are called idioms.

Match the idiom with the corresponding attitude it relates to.

1. _____ Perseverance
2. _____ Honesty/directness
3. _____ Anger
4. _____ Hard work
5. _____ Kindness and helpfulness
6. _____ Cooperation
7. _____ Compromise
8. _____ Independence
9. _____ Happiness
10. _____ Privacy

a. give and take
b. work like a dog
c. hang in there
d. on top of the world
e. cut the apron strings
f. lay your cards on the table
g. two heads are better than one
h. give you the shirt off my back
i. breathing space
j. hot-headed

Answers can be found in Appendix F.

Finally, enthusiasm for learning and performing the task at hand is important. This does not mean you are enthusiastic because someone is dying, and you have to perform cardiopulmonary resuscitation (CPR). Rather, you accept the reality of the situation, and because you have trained well, you are enthusiastic to save a life. Enthusiasm shows as an eagerness or excitement for what you are doing. It helps make the learning go easier. It also helps present a positive attitude. Enthusiasm is a highly contagious condition that is worth getting.

Professional Image

Although you may not be aware of it, your reputation—the image other people have about you—begins the first moment that you walk into a room. You never get a second chance to make a first impression. Think of when you or a loved one was treated by medical professionals. What were the characteristics of the people you believed were professional? Were there any contacts that were unprofessional? Let us explore the attitudes that would lead to a professional reputation.

Skill Application 2–4 **Professional Attitudes**

1. Describe a situation in which a person's attitude made a difficult situation easier for you.

_____

_____

2. Why is it important to be tactful when dealing with others?

_____

_____

3. How would you gain the trust of a skeptical or withdrawn patient?

_____

_____

_____

Skill Application 2–5 **Taking a Look at Yourself**

Let us explore some of the characteristics that can enhance your professional image. We talk more about how to take care of yourself in upcoming chapters, but we can begin to get a baseline as to where you are now. Check the items you think you do on a regular basis. Your goal should be to eventually have all the items checked.

1. _____ I take quiet time to clear my mind and recharge my batteries.

2. _____ I take pride in my work.

3. _____ I am on time for school/work.

4. _____ I avoid using slang or jargon terms in conversation.

5. _____ I work on my conversational skills and attempt to enhance my vocabulary.

6. _____ I present proper body language when interacting with others (listen genuinely, make direct eye contact, avoid fidgeting around or tapping my foot or looking at my watch).

7. _____ I do not smoke or chew gum.

8. _____ I dress professionally (clothes are clean, well pressed, and well fitted). The trendy, casual look is good in school, but a more formal professional look is needed on your job and will assist you in commanding the authority you need to deliver health care.

9. _____ I smile and am pleasant to be with.

10. _____ I do not complain all the time.

(continues)

(continued)

11. _____ I show a genuine interest in others.

12. _____ I make others feel important by respecting their ideas and giving praise when it is due.

13. _____ I acknowledge other points of view and am willing to change ideas and behaviors when necessary.

14. _____ I am a good listener and I do not gossip.

15. _____ I do not brag or act superior.

16. _____ I accept responsibility for my mistakes and try to correct them.

Positive and Negative Attitudes

Your attitude influences how you think and feel about life. This in turn determines your behaviors and how well you interact or get along with others. You have two choices. Do you want to have a positive or negative attitude (Figure 2–5)?

In less than 30 seconds, you have made an impression on others. A first impression is the opinion that others make about you because of the image you present. If your first impression is positive, they will probably want to get to know you. So what will you present?

Is the glass half-empty or half-full? Is the weather partly sunny or partly cloudy? Is this going to be a good day or a bad day? What would you pick? Your answer depends on your attitude. A person with a positive attitude would say the glass is half-full, it is a partly sunny day, and the day is going to be good. Realistically, things may happen that may not make it a perfect day, but a positive person will make the best of it, maintaining a **positive attitude** and being upbeat, optimistic, and cheerful, even in the face of adversity. The positive person will enjoy the day and be excited about what they are doing. Others will enjoy being around that person. With a positive attitude, you will convey the three professional attitudes

Figure 2–5
Do you have a positive or a negative attitude?

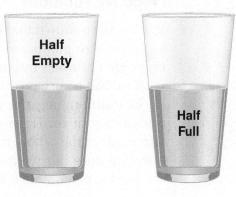

discussed previously. This will put patients at ease and help them in their recovery process. In addition, your coworkers will enjoy working with you.

However, a person with a **negative attitude** will see a half-empty glass and be angry about the partly cloudy day. This attitude conveys unhappiness and is not very pleasant to be around. Pessimists will be sure it is going to be a bad day and will complain often and blame others for their misery. Is this the type of person you would want to spend time with?

Positive Attitudes

Thinking positively can enhance every aspect of your life. It could be one of the most important attitudes that will relate to your success. However, learning to think positively is like learning to do anything else—it takes knowledge and practice.

So what are some of the characteristics of a person with a positive attitude? We already discussed many of them. A willingness to learn and accept changes, enthusiasm, and respect for others. A positive outlook on life shows through in your body language. A friendly facial expression reflects a positive attitude. It also shows that you are calm and in control of the situation.

Positive people are also open to others' viewpoints and backgrounds. This means being able to at least consider new ideas, opinions, and different cultural backgrounds. You may not agree, but you listen and do not judge the individual. Most people would agree that this is how they would want to be treated. This willingness to be open is also a sign of your maturity and flexibility.

Positive people accept responsibility and constructive criticism. They admit their mistakes without blaming others or making excuses. Positive people can do the things necessary to correct their errors and learn how to avoid repeating them.

Positive people also have a good sense of humor. Humor is important in health care for many reasons. It helps the healing process for many patients. It also helps relieve the stress of many tense situations that can occur in the hospital environment. However, humor must be used at the appropriate time and place or it could also be offensive.

Negative Attitudes

Studies have shown that the average child receives 432 negative messages per day, compared with 32 positive. Many contend these messages are absorbed into our subconscious, internalized, and carried with us. Not a very positive thought.

In addition, negative attitudes can be quite contagious and cause others to join in. Have you ever heard the expression, "One bad apple spoils the whole barrel"? A person with a negative attitude is one who does not welcome change or accept imperfections in others. Such a person often blames others for their "bad" situation. This type of person is not very pleasant to work with because they always have a complaint about someone or something. Having a complaint about a situation is okay. However, a negative person will not offer any positive solutions, yet may continue to stir up the problem. A positive person will properly state the problem and think of ways to make it better.

Skill Application 2–6 Positive Attitudes

1. What positive attitudes do you find appealing? Why?

_____

_____

2. What are your favorite songs and TV shows? Do many of them have positive messages?

_____

_____

3. List 10 positive things about yourself. Jot down the first things that come to mind; these are usually your truest feelings. Make sure they are just what you think is wonderful about you, not what others think.

a. _____   f. _____

b. _____   g. _____

c. _____   h. _____

d. _____   i. _____

e. _____   j. _____

4. Make a star by the top three you would want to be remembered by. Now think about qualities you did not list. Now pick two professional qualities you want to work on and describe how you will work on these.

_____

_____

Had we asked you to list your negatives, would this list have been easier to make? If so, you are not alone, but you must work on breaking the negative cycle.

Victim Attitude

The book *The Oz Principle*, by Connors, Smith, and Hickman, states America is in crisis because of a **victim attitude**. It goes on to state that this attitude, which perpetuates helplessness, keeps the person in that victim mode. Granted many people have bad situations, but

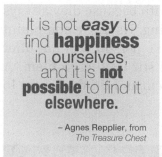

It is not *easy* to find **happiness** in ourselves, and it is **not possible** to find it elsewhere.

– Agnes Repplier, from *The Treasure Chest*

Figure 2–6
You must create your own happiness.

there is hope for change. You do not need to call a psychic hot line for the answer. The solution lies within yourself (Figure 2–6).

The Oz Principle states four steps to get out of the victim mode. They are:

See it: Identify the problem.

Own it: Take personal responsibility for it.

Solve it: Identify possible options.

Do it: Pick an option and take action to implement it.

One suggestion would be to add "check it: assess the outcome" to this list as the final step. In other words, evaluate your solution to see how effective it is and modify it accordingly. The Reverend Jesse Jackson, a civil rights leader who grew up in poverty, achieved many great accomplishments because of his belief in the power of a person's attitude. He stated: "I am somebody! If my mind can conceive it, and my heart can believe it, I know I can achieve it!"

Changing Negative Attitudes into Positive Attitudes

There are other ways to change negative attitudes into positive. Have you ever heard of a *self-fulfilling prophecy*? It means if you believe something strongly enough, it can come true.

For example, if you tell yourself that you will never get organized, you will not. However, you can use this same principle to your advantage by using positive self-talk. Talking to yourself does not mean you are crazy. In fact, talking is slower than thinking and, therefore, slows your racing mind down. This allows you to be more focused.

Self-talk can boost self-esteem if it is optimistic and positive. Replace negative internal messages such as "I'm not smart enough," with "If I study hard I *can* do well." Do not dwell on past negative or unpleasant experiences and do not carry grudges. This only depletes your energy and destroys motivation.

Be open and direct with your communications. And remember to lighten up and take care of yourself.

Food **for** Thought 2–3

Timeless Wisdom
The fault, dear Brutus, is not in our stars, but in ourselves.

—Shakespeare, *Julius Caesar*

What was William Shakespeare trying to convey?

_____

_____

Food **for** Thought 2–4

Humor in Medicine
LAUGHTER is contagious . . . start an epidemic.
—Author Unknown

It may seem strange to talk about humor in the medical professions. However, much scientific research is now being done to determine the benefits of humor in the healing process. Some research suggests that laughter helps the immune system become better in warding off illness (Figure 2–7). This is not to say that humor therapy and positive emotions can replace medical treatment. They simply can enhance the medical treatment and the body's positive response. Let's look at the process of laughter.

A good laugh has been shown to increase the heart rate and improve blood circulation. Epinephrine levels in the blood also rise. This is the body's arousal hormone and stimulates the release of **endorphins**. Endorphins are the body's natural painkillers. In addition, other **immunologic**

"Smile, people will wonder what you're up to!"

Figure 2–7
Smiling and laughter are good for the soul.

responses are increased. Finally, the entire respiratory system gets a workout along with our facial muscles. These are some physiologic outcomes of laughter, but what about the psychological effects?

Humor has been shown to relieve tension and lessen anxiety. This is important in the sometimes frightening hospital environment. Humor can also help self-image and stimulate creativity when appropriately used. Some smoking cessation programs are now using humor therapy to help substitute humor as a coping strategy for the addictive and dangerous nicotine. In Chapter 1, you were encouraged to use humor in making up silly stories to aid your learning. So use humor when you can, and remember that what is learned with humor is not readily forgotten. To help you, we have included some fictitious mixed-up medical terminologies.

Cesarean section: a district in Rome

Coma: a punctuation mark

Dilate: to live long

Fester: quicker

GI series: baseball games between teams of soldiers

Medical staff: a physician's cane

Morbid: a higher offer

Outpatient: a person who has fainted

Protein: in favor of young people

Serology: study of English knighthood

Tumor: an extra pair

Urine: opposite of you're out

Varicose veins: veins that are very close together

Finally, remember that no one is perfect. For example, many people view anger as a negative emotion. However, a little anger can be good. It spurs us on to do better or to right an injustice. Another example is that we all feel sad when tragedy strikes. This is what makes us human. However, taken to extremes, anger can be dangerous and sadness can lead to severe depression.

An important idea to think about is that people do not get you upset, you do! You are the only person who can make you angry or upset or feel bad. *You* feel the way *you* think.

Skill Application 2–7 Using Positive Self-Talk

Complete the following statements with examples of positive self-talk.

Example

When I realize I have made a mistake, I tell myself that *it is okay, everyone makes a mistake. The important thing is to learn from my mistakes, move on, and improve.* This is an example of positive self-talk. An example of negative self-talk would be "I am so dumb, I never get anything right."

1. When I am criticized, I . . .

2. When nothing I do seems to be right, I . . .

3. When I do something good, I . . .

4. When I get angry, I . . .

5. When I do something that I think is wrong, I . . .

6. When I have a good idea, I . . .

7. When I feel anxious about something, I . . .

What negative attitudes bother you the most? Why?

_____

_____

Just For FUN 2-2

Descriptive Attitudes

Here are some attitudes that you do not want to be associated with.

The tank: confrontational and aggressive

The sniper: identifies everyone's weakness and talks behind others' backs

The grenade: explodes suddenly about things that have nothing to do with the circumstances

(continues)

(continued)

The know-it-all: seldom in doubt, has low tolerance for anyone who disagrees with them, and if something goes wrong, it was somebody else's fault

The yes person: quick to agree, slow to deliver—unkept commitments and broken promises but always says yes to please

The maybe person: puts off decisions till it's too late—never commits

The no person: deadly to morale, able to defeat great ideas in a single syllable—discouraging

The whiner: overwhelmed by an unfair world—no one measures up to their standard of perfection

The denier: says there is no problem—ignore or deny it and it will go away

Food **for** Thought 2–5

You Can Make a Difference
The following story is an example of someone making a difference.

The Starfish
There was a young man walking down a deserted beach just before dawn. In the distance he saw a frail old man. As he approached the old man, he saw him picking up stranded starfish and throwing them back into the sea. The young man gazed in wonder as the old man again and again threw the small starfish from the sand to the water. He asked him, "Why do you spend so much energy doing what seems to be a waste of time?" The old man explained that the stranded starfish would die if left in the morning sun. "But there must be thousands of beaches and millions of starfish," exclaimed the young man. "How can your effort make any difference?" The old man looked down at the small starfish in his hand and as he threw it to safety in the sea said, "It makes a difference to this one."

What does this story mean to you? Remember you have one precious chance called a lifetime. It is up to you to make the most of every day. Celebrate and be enthusiastic about life. If you make a positive difference in just one person's life, you have done well. Think of how many lives you can touch as a health care professional! (Figure 2–8)

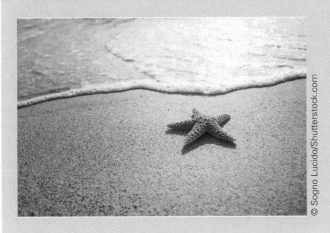

© Sogno Lucido/Shutterstock.com

Figure 2–8
You can and do make a difference!

Showcasing Your Academic Performance and Professionalism

The search for your ideal career or the ideal path in life begins not when you graduate, but on the first day of your academic program. You will spend much of your academic career building your résumé or portfolio, networking, and showcasing yourself in a positive manner. You want to build skills that will enable you to obtain that first great career position. Good grades are not the only ingredient that factors into getting a good job when you graduate. Your extracurricular activities, volunteerism, attendance, and enthusiasm for learning all play a role in creating your own personal **brand**. A personal brand is a type of marketing tool that includes in-person elements and online elements. As stated in Chapter 1, the authors prefer the term *showcase* as it implies a more authentic or truer image, and therefore, we are interweaving it with the term *brand*. Showcasing includes in-person and online elements. In-person elements include the way you act, talk, dress, and spend your time. The online elements include how you act, talk, and present yourself online. These items will set you apart from others in either a positive or negative way.

Perhaps the best way to explain this concept is by looking at two student examples. Both students are seeking an entry-level position upon graduation in a durable medical equipment (DME) company.

Susan has a 2.8 grade point average (GPA). She has struggled some with her classes and has averaged a B or B+. She makes sure to always attend class and any extra study sessions. She holds a part-time job as a work study at her college library. In addition, she is involved in two campus organizations, one that focuses on her major and the other that is a service organization. Susan makes time to volunteer for community service projects for each of the organizations and makes sure to keep track of those hours. During her junior year, she is elected the president of the organization focused on her major and helps to organize a successful peer mentoring program. She links this program to her online social media accounts and makes sure to post pictures of her volunteer activities. Susan limits her involvement to these two organizations and her schoolwork.

James is a successful student; he has made the dean's list every semester and has a 3.7 GPA. He maintains a part-time job in food service in a community adjacent to his college. He has not joined any organizations or clubs on campus because he is just too busy studying. He has been approached by instructors and other students to help tutor students; however, he always declines. He misses class on occasion to study for other upcoming exams and does not attend study sessions, since he would rather study alone. He often posts negative comments on his social media sites and allows friends to identify him in unflattering pictures.

Both students have strengths and weaknesses. Arguments could be made that either of them has the advantage. However, Susan has showcased herself as a student who is giving and committed to her community as well as a team player. Her personal brand is one that most employers would be thrilled to have join their organization.

Skill Application 2–8 **Showcasing Yourself Early**

Think about the students Susan and James described earlier.

Which student has the stronger academic record? _____

Which student has a personal brand that identifies them as helpful and committed to the community? _____

List three strengths of each student.

_____

_____

_____

List three weaknesses of each student.

_____

_____

_____

Food **for** Thought 2–6

Good Habits

Good habits are the ways of behaving that are acceptable and beneficial to an individual or society. Some good habits you may already practice are as follows:

Being respectful to others

Respecting the environment

Attending school regularly

Completing assigned tasks properly and on time

Being friendly to a newcomer in your neighborhood or class

Being honest in all your activities and responsibilities

Not smoking or chewing gum

Taking care of yourself with good nutrition and exercise

(continues)

(continued)

> *Bad habits* are those behaviors that are annoying or unacceptable to individuals or society. Do you have any bad habits that you need to work on? Remember, the best way to break a bad habit is to drop it.
>
> One bad habit that causes a lot of grief is gossip. Gossip can wreck marriages, ruin reputations, and cause heartaches. Before you repeat a negative story about someone, ask yourself: Is it true? Is it fair? Is it necessary?
>
> List three *good* habits you want to develop.
>
> _____
>
> _____
>
> _____

Skill Application 2–9 First Impressions

In less than 30 seconds, you have made an impression on others. A first impression is the opinion that others make about you as a result of the image that you present at your introduction. If your first impression is positive, others will probably want to get to know you.

1. How do first impressions affect your patient interaction?

   _____

   _____

2. List five things you can do to make a positive first impression with a patient or a coworker (for example, a smile and a firm handshake).

   a. _____

   b. _____

   c. _____

   d. _____

   e. _____

Summary

- A high degree of professionalism must be maintained in the health care professions. Good self-motivation and self-esteem are key ingredients in achieving professionalism.
- Self-esteem is shaped by your values or what you believe. To be successful, you must begin with good self-esteem and a set of positive values and attitudes. There are certain attitudes required of a health care professional that are listed as follows:
- This chapter will help you contrast positive and negative attitudes and develop personal action plans to

enhance professionalism and positive attitudes.

- A trustworthy attitude develops from being honest, dependable, and responsible.
- A caring attitude is fostered by showing sincerity, empathy, respect, and tact when dealing with patients and coworkers.
- A competent attitude will be demonstrated by your enthusiasm and willingness to learn and accept change, coupled with acceptance of proper criticism.
- A personal positive attitude will greatly influence your future success as a health care professional.
- A self-confident attitude that can advocate for patient care and safety.
- Developing a personal brand early in your academic career will "showcase" your academic and personal achievements and this in turn will help your career potential later.

Case Study 2–1

John was a new health care professional in the office. During his orientation, he presented a know-it-all attitude with his coworkers who were attempting to help him become comfortable in his new position. He was very aggressive (not assertive) and in a loud and sarcastic voice pointed out all the things wrong in the office. In addition, he went on about where he had worked before and how they had done everything right. Although his coworkers pressed him for specific examples for improvement, he really did not have any. He was appropriately told about his attitude and the potential for problems if it continued. Within 3 months, he left the job because "he could not get along with coworkers or patients." In addition, he made several errors with his patients.

Do you think his aggressive know-it-all attitude was a cover for a very insecure individual, or do you have other possible explanations?

_____

_____

_____

How would you characterize John's handling of constructive criticism?

_____

_____

_____

What specific attitudes does John need to develop before going on to his next position?

_____

_____

_____

Without taking the steps to change, what do you think John's future work record will demonstrate?

_____

_____

_____

Internet Activity   Using Internet search engines, try to find additional material on personal and professional characteristics for success that you can share with your fellow students. Some suggested keywords are professionalism, branding, self-motivation, lifelong learning, positive thinking, and positive attitudes. Write down something new to share.

_____

_____

_____

Chapter 3

Setting Goals and Time Management

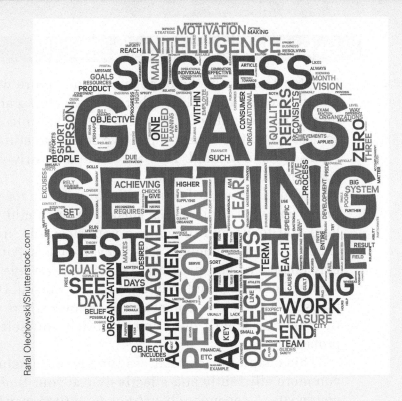

Rafal Olechowski/Shutterstock.com

Objectives

Upon completion of this chapter, you should be able to:

1. Set effective personal, educational, career, and community goals.

2. Differentiate between long-, medium-, and short-range goals.

3. Develop action plans to achieve *your* stated goals.

4. Assess your time management skills.

5. Develop effective time management skills.

6. Identify time-wasting habits.

7. Correct time-wasting habits.

Key Terms

goal	**objective**	**short-range goal**
long-range goal	**plateau period**	**time management skill**
medium-range goal	**procrastination**	**visualization**

Introduction

Whoever wants to reach a distant goal must take many small steps.

—Helmut Schmidt

Chapter 2 gave you the opportunity to explore who you are. This chapter begins to explore where you are going and how you plan on getting there. It is important to note that professionals with high self-esteem not only have a positive confident attitude but also walk with a mission in mind. They are continually striving to achieve their goals or visions.

Learning to set goals creates the foundation for your professional image and your professional success. You should use your goals to help you focus and to achieve your desired "brand" early. This chapter shows you how to set achievable goals. Although your goals may change as you progress, you should always have the goal of seeking knowledge and striving to better yourself. Having solid goals that showcase you as someone who knows where they are heading in their career will help you establish yourself in your chosen profession.

This chapter also discusses time management. This will help you more efficiently and effectively use your time to help achieve your goals. A secondary benefit of good time management is that it will *free up* more time for you to enjoy yourself. All work and no play is not good. You must also nurture yourself and have fun. Time management will help you accomplish this task. In turn, this will make you feel better about yourself and become more committed to your goals. It all fits together.

Setting goals will be part of your everyday activities as a health care professional. You will need to develop therapeutic goals and treatment plans for your patients. In addition, in the hectic health care environment, good time management skills are a must.

Put "the initial time" in on this chapter. Once these techniques become a part of your everyday life, it will save you a great deal of time and make you much more productive. It will also make your life much more enjoyable.

Anticipatory Exercise 3–1 **What Are Your Goals?**

Do you normally set goals? _____

If so, what kind of goals? _____

On a scale of 1–10 with 10 being the best, rate yourself as a time manager. _____

Describe where you see yourself in 1 year.

_____

_____

Describe where you see yourself in 3 years.

_____

_____

Setting Goals

Developing **goals** will help you decide where you want to go. But what are goals? Goals are specific accomplishments you aim to achieve. There is a common acronym for these types of goals, it is SMART. SMART stands for Specific, Measurable, Achievable, Relevant, and Time-based. Effective goals should have five major characteristics, as shown in Figure 3–1. Effective goals should be:

- Specific and Self-chosen
- Measurable
- Achievable
- Relevant
- Time-based and positive

Figure 3–1
Goals—the foundations upon which to live your life.

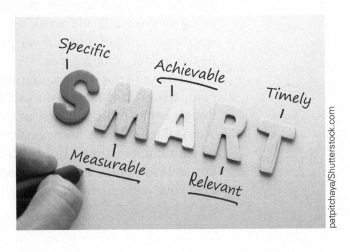

patpitchaya/Shutterstock.com

Specific and Self-Chosen

The "S" stands for specific and we will help you develop specific goals shortly. However, we are also adding another "S" in Self-chosen. There may be several well-meaning people in your life who might try to set goals for you. Although you should consider what they have to say, you must ultimately choose your own goals. This gives you ownership and responsibility for your goals. Your goals should be something *you* desire and really want to do. Have you ever heard stories of patients who "willed" themselves to die? Even though the health care professional's goal was to treat them and make them better, this was not the patient's Self-chosen goal. Another example is choosing a career. Do you know someone (even yourself?) who was pressured into choosing a college major by their parent or guardian? They may go through the motions of attending college, but may be very unhappy or unsuccessful.

Measurable

Your goal must be specific and measurable. For example, let us say that your goal is to "do well in your health sciences courses." This is too vague. How well is well? If you state that your goal is to "get a B or better in each of your health sciences courses," you now have a measure of your success. You will know for sure if you have achieved the goal or not.

Achievable

You must be able to see yourself (conceive of) accomplishing the goal. You must be able to believe you can do it. Remember, if you conceive it and believe it, you can achieve it. If you set the goal of winning a talent show, but never enter, you will never win. Another way to say this is that the goal must be realistic.

Relevant

The goal should also be relevant. It should be related to something you are actively working on. Don't set a goal of being an NFL quarterback if you have never played football. Your goal should also be moderately challenging.

Consider sports, for example; it may be easy to play against weak competition and make yourself look really good. However, you will not get better until you play against strong competition and challenge yourself to improve. Many coaches will tell you "You are only as good as your competition." In health care, you must constantly challenge yourself to obtain new knowledge, skills, and attitudes in order to give your patients the most current and best treatments.

Time-Based and Positive

It is also very important to set a time period for completion and always use positive language when stating a goal. One goal that a group of health care professionals developed was to "increase physician interactions." However, this can mean more conflicts between physicians and this would indeed satisfy the goal of more interactions. The new goal should then become "to increase positive physician interactions."

Objectives

Objectives are related to goals. Objectives are things you need to do in order to achieve your stated goal. Objectives can also be thought of as the specific steps in your overall action plan to realize your goal. Developing specific objectives and action plans will ensure that you reach your goal.

For example, your goal may be to become a physical therapist specializing in sports medicine for a professional basketball team. You must now develop an action plan comprising specific objectives that will help you reach this goal. Some of the objectives may include researching the degree requirements and talking to physical therapists.

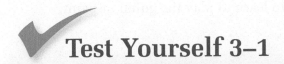 **Test Yourself 3–1**

Which Is a Better Goal?
Choose the better goal statement in each pair.

1. a. I will do better with my patients and try to be more helpful.
   b. I will assess my patient interaction skills and develop action plans to improve them.

2. a. I will exercise three times a week.
   b. I will get in better shape so that I look better at the beach.

3. a. I will successfully pass the cardiopulmonary resuscitation (CPR) course.
   b. I may take a CPR course, if it is not too hard.

4. a. I will do volunteer work with older adults to improve my skills with geriatric patients.
   b. I will try to get to know older people better.

5. a. I will change my eating habits to maintain a weight of 150 lbs.
   b. I will not eat junk food.

Answers can be found in Appendix F.

Types of Goals

There are several types of goals. Goals can be broken down into specific categories to allow you to focus on the various aspects of your life. This text focuses on the following categories of goals:

- Career/professional goals
- Personal goals
- Educational goals
- Community goals

Career/Professional Goals

These are the goals related to obtaining the career of your choice. Once you obtain your career, you can then make specific professional goals to improve your knowledge and skills so that you can be the best health care provider in your chosen health profession.

Personal Goals

You may have personal goals, such as to improve your self-esteem or a relationship with someone. You may also want to improve your physical well-being. These goals can include learning a new skill or hobby. Perhaps you want to learn to play the guitar or paint.

Educational Goals

You may have educational goals such as completing this year with a B+ average. However, these are not just school-related goals. For example, a goal may be to learn a new technique such as CPR, first aid, another language, or sign language. All of these would help complement your health professional skills. These are goals that will help showcase your academic success and professionalism.

Community Goals

We are all part of a community. Becoming involved in your community can help improve neighborhood conditions. In addition, it will give you valuable skills and experience and may help you make contacts that will be beneficial to your future. This is definitely a win-win situation. This means you win, or gain benefit, from this interaction, and your community wins by being improved. These goals may include volunteer work with people who are homeless or older adults. Another goal may be coaching children in your community or teaching adults how to read. These goals will help you to focus on your desire to be showcased as a compassionate, community-minded individual.

It is important to achieve a balance with your types of goals. If you have all educational goals and no personal development goals, you may soon "burn out" from not taking care of yourself. Your educational goals may then suffer. So develop a balance of goals that will complement each other and lead to your focus as someone who knows where they are going.

Goals can also be broken down according to the time frame in which they will be accomplished. You can have **short-**, **medium-**, or **long-range goals**.

- Short range: to be accomplished tomorrow, next week, next month
- Medium range: to be accomplished within the next 6 months or 1 year
- Long range: to be accomplished within the next 3–5 years

Short- and medium-range goals are needed to accomplish your long-range goals, as illustrated in Figure 3–2.

Figure 3–2
Obtaining long-range goals.

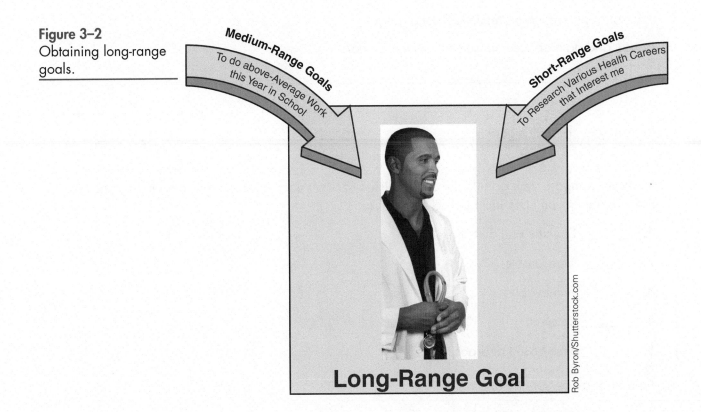

Medium-Range Goals
To do above-Average Work this Year in School

Short-Range Goals
To Research Various Health Careers that Interest me

Long-Range Goal

Rob Byron/Shutterstock.com

Skill Application 3–1 Developing and Refining Long-Range Goals

This chapter states that goals should be:

- Specific and Self-chosen
- Measurable
- Achievable
- Relevant
- Time-based and positive

Use these criteria to develop a long-range (within 5 years) goal for each of the four types of goals discussed in your text.

Example

Type of goal: *career/professional—long range*

Range and date of accomplishment: *within 5 years*

Your goal: *to graduate with an associate degree from an accredited respiratory therapy school. I will graduate in the top 10% of my class.*

Reason you chose this goal: *I had severe asthma as a child and realize the importance of being able to breathe. I want to make a difference in patients who are fighting for each breath.*

Your Turn

Type of goal: *career/professional—long range*

Range and date of accomplishment: *within 5 years*

Your goal: _____

_____

Reason you chose this goal: _____

_____

Now compare your goal to the criteria list. Check off each criterion and rewrite your statement if needed until you have included all the criteria.

1. _____ Specific and Self-chosen

2. _____ Measurable

3. _____ Achievable

4. _____ Relevant

5. _____ Time-based and positive

Type of goal: *personal—long range*

Range and date of accomplishment: *within 5 years*

(continues)

(continued)

Your goal: _____

_____

Reason you chose this goal: _____

_____

    Now compare your goal to the criteria list. Check off each criterion and rewrite your statement if needed until you have included all the criteria.

1. _____ Specific and Self-chosen

2. _____ Measurable

3. _____ Achievable

4. _____ Relevant

5. _____ Time-based and positive

Type of goal: *educational—long range*

Range and date of accomplishment: *within 5 years*

Your goal: _____

_____

Reason you chose this goal: _____

_____

    Now compare your goal to the criteria list. Check off each criterion and rewrite your statement if needed until you have included all the criteria.

1. _____ Specific and Self-chosen

2. _____ Measurable

3. _____ Achievable

4. _____ Relevant

5. _____ Time-based and positive

Type of goal: *community—long range*

Range and date of accomplishment: *within 5 years*

Your goal: _____

_____

Reason you chose this goal: _____

_____

(continues)

(continued)

Now compare your goal to the criteria list. Check off each criterion and rewrite your statement if needed until you have included all the criteria.

1. _____ Specific and Self-chosen

2. _____ Measurable

3. _____ Achievable

4. _____ Relevant

5. _____ Time-based and positive

Skill Application 3–2 Refining Long-Range Goals

Now, rewrite each of the previous goals to include an action plan that contains specific objectives and resources that will help you in your quest.

Example

Type of goal: *career/professional—long range*

Range and date of accomplishment: *within 5 years*

Your goal: *to graduate with an associate degree from an accredited respiratory therapy school. I will graduate in the top 10% of my class.*

Reason you chose this goal: *I had severe asthma as a child and realize the importance of being able to breathe. I want to make a difference in patients who are fighting for each breath. I want to showcase myself as a quality health care provider who strives to achieve excellence as demonstrated by my academic and professional achievements.*

Action plan (specific objectives):

1. *Investigate the field of respiratory care and determine requirements.*

2. *Do "B" work or better in my health science courses to get accepted to the program.*

3. *Do volunteer work and get to know some future contacts within the profession.*

Resources to help achieve: *my health science teachers, local hospital, library, local community college, and my determination to succeed.*

Your Goals and Action Plans

Type of goal: *career/professional—long range*

Range and date of accomplishment: _____

Your goal: _____

_____

(continues)

(continued)

Reason you chose this goal: _____

_____

Action plan (specific objectives):

1. _____

2. _____

3. _____

Resources to help achieve it: _____

_____

Type of goal: *personal—long range*

Range and date of accomplishment: _____

Your goal: _____

_____

Reason you chose this goal: _____

_____

Action plan (specific objectives):

1. _____

2. _____

3. _____

Resources to help achieve it: _____

_____

Type of goal: *educational—long range*

Range and date of accomplishment: _____

Your goal: _____

_____

Reason you chose this goal: _____

_____

Action plan (specific objectives):

1. _____

2. _____

3. _____

(continues)

(continued)

Resources to help achieve it: _____

_____

Type of goal: *community—long range*

Range and date of accomplishment: _____

Your goal: _____

_____

Reason you chose this goal: _____

_____

Action plan (specific objectives):

1. _____

2. _____

3. _____

Resources to help achieve it: _____

_____

Skill Application 3–3 Developing Short- and Medium-Range Goals

Now that you have completed your long-term goals, you have your vision. You are not going to achieve this overnight. You must now take small steps in your journey. You must develop short- and medium-range goals to achieve your long-range goals. For each of your long-range goals, write one short-term (accomplished within a month) and one medium-term (accomplished within 6 months) goal that will complement your long-range goal and move you toward it.

Type of goal: *career/professional—short term*

Range and date of accomplishment: _____

Your goal: _____

_____

Reason you chose this goal: _____

_____

(continues)

(continued)

Action plan (specific objectives):

1. _____

2. _____

3. _____

Resources to help achieve it: _____

_____

Type of goal: *career/professional—medium term*

Range and date of accomplishment: _____

Your goal: _____

_____

Reason you chose this goal: _____

_____

Action plan (specific objectives):

1. _____

2. _____

3. _____

Resources to help achieve it: _____

_____

Type of goal: *personal—short term*

Range and date of accomplishment: _____

Your goal: _____

_____

Reason you chose this goal: _____

_____

Action plan (specific objectives):

1. _____

2. _____

3. _____

Resources to help achieve it: _____

_____

(continues)

(continued)

Type of goal: *personal—medium term*

Range and date of accomplishment: _____

Your goal: _____

_____

Reason you chose this goal: _____

_____

Action plan (specific objectives):

1. _____

2. _____

3. _____

Resources to help achieve it: _____

_____

Type of goal: *educational—short term*

Range and date of accomplishment: _____

Your goal: _____

_____

Reason you chose this goal: _____

_____

Action plan (specific objectives):

1. _____

2. _____

3. _____

Resources to help achieve it: _____

_____

Type of goal: *educational—medium term*

Range and date of accomplishment: _____

Your goal: _____

_____

Reason you chose this goal: _____

_____

(continues)

(continued)

Action plan (specific objectives):

1. _____

2. _____

3. _____

Resources to help achieve it: _____

_____

Type of goal: *community—short term*

Range and date of accomplishment: _____

Your goal: _____

_____

Reason you chose this goal: _____

_____

Action plan (specific objectives):

1. _____

2. _____

3. _____

Resources to help achieve it: _____

_____

Type of goal: *community—medium term*

Range and date of accomplishment: _____

Your goal: _____

_____

Reason you chose this goal: _____

_____

Action plan (specific objectives):

1. _____

2. _____

3. _____

Resources to help achieve it: _____

_____

Food for Thought 3–1

The United States Olympic Training Program

The United States Olympic Committee has developed a training program to have their athletes "think" like winners. It includes the following four main components:

- Visualize yourself in the successful performance of your event.
- Set short- and long-term goals to achieve "the gold."
- Practice physical and mental relaxation techniques.
- Concentrate on positive thoughts.

How does this relate to what you have learned so far? How does it apply to your life? What about your future health care career?

Helpful Hints on Goal Setting

One hint is to prioritize your goals so that you get a timeline of when they need to be accomplished. Remember, when changes occur you may need to reprioritize your goals or develop new objectives.

Visualization can also help you reach your goal. Visualize what it will be like when you have reached your goal. Picture and feel all the good feelings. This will help you maintain your commitment.

Many people start out "full force" toward a goal for a short while and then taper off. This is natural. At first you may make rapid progress toward a goal. Eventually, you may reach a period when this progress stalls. This is called a **plateau period**, where you see little or no progress toward your goal. This is the crucial stage in which you should not give up! Realize that everyone reaches this plateau period and that it will pass.

Finally, talk to other people who have achieved the goal you are working toward. Find out what they did. Learn from their mistakes. They may also prove to be valuable contacts in the future.

Time Management

To think too long about doing a thing often becomes its undoing.

—Eva Young

Someone once said that time is life. Therefore, if you waste time, you are actually wasting your life. However, be careful not to take this view too far. Taking a walk in the woods may be considered by some to be a waste of time, but it is not. Taking that walk may give you time to clear your mind, recharge your batteries, or just enjoy the beauty of nature. This certainly is time well spent. However, balance is the key. If you always walk in the woods and do not do the things you need to do in your life, it can have serious consequences.

It is best to think of time as a nonrenewable resource. Therefore, use it wisely. You may have heard of the saying "carpe diem," which is Latin for seize the day. But to truly be an effective time manager and to live life to its fullest, you should "seize the moment."

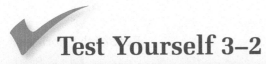

Test Yourself 3–2

Do You Need to Be a Better Time Manager?

Check the following items that relate to you:

1. _____ I complain about lack of time or say there is not enough time in the day.

2. _____ I put things off until the last minute.

3. _____ I get stressed out when given a large assignment.

4. _____ Deadlines make me anxious.

5. _____ I am often late for appointments or turning in assignments.

6. _____ I get overwhelmed with a task and do not know where to start.

7. _____ I spend long periods of time texting, playing with apps, or social media.

8. _____ I jump from one task to another.

If you checked one or two items, you are a good time manager and can work on only those areas. If you checked three or four items, you are fair and could use some help. If you checked five or six, you are a poor time manager and would greatly benefit from this chapter. If you checked seven or eight, it means that if you follow through with the suggestions and work in this chapter, it will be a positive life-changing experience.

Using Time Management Techniques

Where do you start? The good news is that you have already started. Establishing goals and priorities is the first and best place to start. Goals tell us what is important and the priorities help us focus our energy on the more urgent issues.

Now that you have goals and priorities established, you can assess your time use. You can then develop plans and use tools and techniques to optimize your **time management skills**. Figure 3–3 shows the relationship between goals and time management.

To become an effective time manager, you must look at three areas:

- Minimize the "time wasters" in your life.
- Make effective lists.
- Capitalize on your personal peak periods of productivity.

Figure 3–3
The whole picture: how goals and effective time management are integrate.

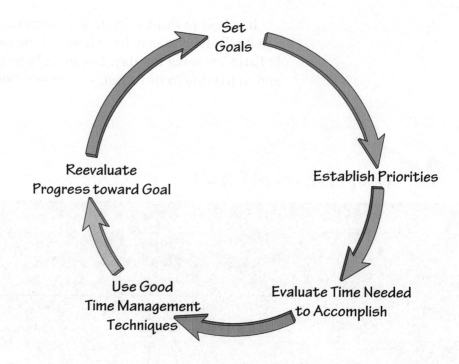

Minimize Time Wasters

Have you ever heard someone say "there aren't enough hours in the day"? Well, the truth is everyone has 24 hours in a day. If you know of a place that has more, many people will want to move there. Seriously, we all have the same amount of time. How we use our time is what makes the difference. One of the first assessment techniques is to identify "common time wasters" that could free up valuable time for other pursuits. On the following pages are listings of common time wasters.

Failure to Plan and Establish Priorities. Without a plan, you have no sense of direction and can wander aimlessly. This wastes time.

You may say, "Yeah, but it takes time to plan!" This is certainly true, but the small amount of time invested in the plan can free up the tremendous amount of time you would waste without it. Part of the plan has to include priorities. You will be working on this soon, but let us give you one example.

Say you had six patients requiring therapy during morning rounds, which last from 0730 to 0930. Each therapy takes about 15 minutes, and breakfast trays come at 0800. You cannot do therapies while the patients are eating. Four of your patients are fresh postoperative patients and have nasogastric tubes inserted. This means that they cannot eat. How would you plan and prioritize your morning rounds to give all the patients an effective and timely treatment?

Just For FUN 3-1

Prioritizing Tasks

Let's say you have reached your long-range career goal and are now a hospital staff member (soon to be promoted) working the daylight, or 7 to 3, shift. You have the following tasks to do. Prioritize this list by writing numbers 1 to 10 on the line to the left of the item, indicating which you would do first, second, and so on. The hospital works on military time, so you might have to review or research how that works. It is very simple.

_____ Do afternoon treatment rounds (1300 to 1430).

_____ Research at the library for a report to your medical director due in 2 weeks.

_____ Reserve a conference room for an in-service for your department. This must be done by 1100.

_____ Do morning treatment rounds (0715 to 0915).

_____ Call two home care patients to reschedule appointments for tomorrow.

_____ Fix and calibrate equipment in the utility room. This will take about 1 hour.

_____ Complete billing charges for yesterday—must be done by end of shift and will take about 30 minutes.

_____ Eat lunch with medical equipment salesperson.

_____ Give end-of-shift report to oncoming 1500 to 2300 shift (about 30 minutes).

_____ Scheduled meeting from 0930 to 1000 with department director concerning my upcoming promotion and raise for doing such a professional job.

Note: Answers can be found in Appendix F.

Overplanning and Overorganizing. You can take planning and organizing to the extreme. Again, come back to the very important point that *you must find a balance.* If you put so much time into developing and organizing a plan, you will have little time for doing anything else.

Remember that overorganizing can be a time waster but balanced organizing is critical. Organization is key to managing your time and energy. Keep your work area neat and tidy; put clutter and distractions away. Keep your notebooks, pens, and paper where they can easily be found. Organize your online files into folders, and use naming conventions for your documents that help you find the most current version.

Cellphones. The cellphone is one of the most useful facilitators of communication ever invented. However, many people can let this device completely control their lives and waste a lot of time. We are not saying that talking/texting with your friends is a waste of time. This is important, but again you must strike a balance. To call/text someone you have just seen in school and gossip for hours certainly is not a productive use of time. Using the cellphone for personal matters during work hours has been identified as a major reason for low productivity in health care. Many people feel that it is rude to leave a text message unanswered. You must realize that when working in health care, your personal messaging must wait until you are on a break or off duty (Figure 3–4).

Social media is another way you can waste time, scrolling through your social media on your phone can take up your time. Place limits on your use, and if necessary, turn off your phone or put it in another room.

The Computer. While the computer is a great time-saving device in many applications such as researching topics and writing reports, it can become a time waster if abused. For example, you can spend too much time in chat rooms, tied up with e-mail and instant messages, or playing computer games and not have enough time to get your academic and clinical work done. You should enjoy the computer, but again maintaining balance is the key. If you have difficulty leaving those distractors alone while working, consider setting up a time schedule that allows you short breaks to answer e-mail and text messages. You must stay within your time limit in order for this strategy to work.

Napping and Sleeping Late. Taking a 20- to 30-minute afternoon nap can be invigorating. However, when you let that nap turn into hours or you sleep until noon everyday, you can be wasting time. A good night's rest is important; you need about 8 hours of sleep each night. Keeping regular hours (i.e., bed at 10 pm and wake at 6 am everyday)

Figure 3–4
Be smart with your cell phone use.

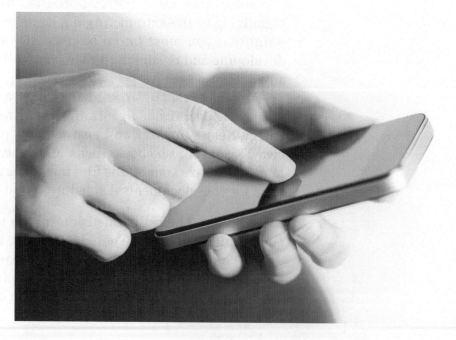

Antlii/Shutterstock.com

can help you. Rising early and getting some tasks done before you start the day (exercising, tidying your work space, or spending some time meditating) can keep you more focused throughout the day.

Personal Habits. Two personal habits that are huge wasters of time are **procrastination** and worry. Procrastination is putting things off until the last minute. Procrastination can be caused by lack of priorities, boredom, anxiety, or fear of failure. It can also be caused by being uncertain about what the task is.

Procrastination and worry are related. Procrastination robs you of time and power by causing stress in the form of guilt, embarrassment, and anxiety. The anxiety and fear of failure can cause worry. Worry is such a powerful enemy of time and causes great stresses on the mind and body that a portion of the next chapter is devoted to it. For now, consider the following: *Many people worry so much about failing that they never accomplish what it was they were worried about.*

Do not procrastinate any longer. Take a look at the list that shows you ways to combat time wasters. And as the famous commercial says, "Just Do It."

Combating Time Wasters: Procrastination and Worry

- Of course, *organize* and *plan.*
- If you are uncertain of what needs to be done, ask!
- Set your priorities so that you are not jumping from one task to another.
- Find ways of making the job interesting. Have fun with what you are doing. Be happy and have a positive attitude.
- Do your most demanding work when you are fresh and alert.
- Reward yourself when you get a job done.
- Organize your desk so that you are not wasting time trying to find pencils, dictionaries, and so on.
- Make use of otherwise down time such as waiting in lines or at the physician's office. Take note cards if you have a doctor's appointment. If you have to wait, instead of getting upset you can use that time to study and that will free up your evening time for some relaxation.
- Take care of yourself! Go to bed a little earlier to recharge your batteries. Get up a half hour sooner to gain productive time. The morning is usually your best and most productive time.
- Control interruptions when doing a task. These can include phone calls and visitors.
- Finish what you start.

Skill Application 3–4 Identifying Time Wasters

Good, effective time management will help you meet deadlines, help you perform better academically, and give you more *free* time. The first step in becoming a good time manager is to identify your time wasters.

Review the list of time wasters in your book. Recopy them here. For 1 week, put a check mark next to each time waster you performed. At the end of the week, see which ones have the most "checks" beside them. Now develop your own goal and action plan to combat your worst time waster habit.

_____

_____

_____

_____

_____

_____

_____

_____

_____

_____

Making Effective Lists

Many successful health care leaders state "making lists" is the secret of their success. This allows them to plan and prioritize their tasks. It also helps them generate ideas and see better ways of combining tasks.

There are several types of lists you can make and several places you can make them. The process of keeping different types of lists can become so confusing that you can become lost in all your lists. Therefore, we recommend a somewhat simpler way to organize your life. The first step is to get the proper tools to help you.

The most important tool is a large desk calendar for your special study area. This can allow you to put all your special upcoming events and deadlines in one place, and at a glance, you can see what your future holds. This type of planning gives you an overview or the entire picture. You can carry a pocket planner or use your phone to mark down things as they come up during the day and then transfer them to your desk calendar.

In the electronic age, handheld computers, smartdevices, and tablets can help you to maintain daily schedules and even produce a calendar of obligations. However, it is important to have something in front of you that shows the "big picture." A store-bought desk calendar or an electronically produced one that you print out facilitates seeing everything at a glance and helps in strategic planning.

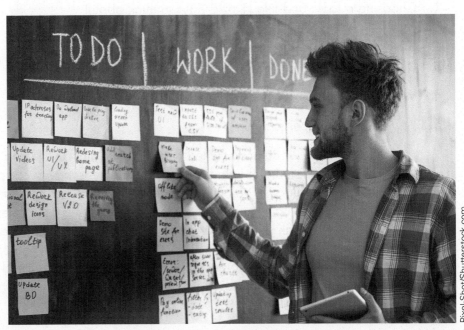

Pixel-Shot/Shutterstock.com

Skill Application 3–5 Working with Your Calendar

If you do not already have one, obtain a large desk calendar and fill in all your commitments, social activities, assignment deadlines, sports activities, and scheduled workdays. Keep it neat. Now take one of your academic deadlines or projects and break it down into manageable steps with approximate times for completion.

List these here and then return to your calendar and place the steps in the appropriate gaps. Make sure you are scheduled to complete the project ahead of your deadline.

Project: _____

Steps: _____

_____

_____

_____

_____

_____

(continues)

(continued)

Now you need to develop more specific plans to meet your deadlines and fulfill your obligations. Pick the major tasks along with their deadlines that are coming up within the next month or so. Now brainstorm and plan all the activities needed to complete the tasks within the deadline. For example, you may have a research paper due in 4 weeks. You would break the task into a logical sequence of events with an approximate time needed to complete each step. This may include the following:

1. Choosing a topic and title (1 or 2 days to think about)

2. Researching and gathering information (10 hours at library)

3. Developing an outline (12 hours)

4. Writing a rough draft (16 hours)

5. Rewriting final paper (6 hours)

You can see from your calendar where you have the time to fill in for each of these tasks. Make sure you give yourself plenty of time before the deadline to have your paper completed. This will provide a buffer zone in case you underestimated the time needed for a certain task or if something unexpected comes up. You can write these tasks on your desk calendar in blocks of time. For example, you might break your library time into 4 days of 2.5 hours each. Remember, your first couple of attempts are learning experiences. Keep records so that you can improve. Now that you have your major tasks planned, you can continue to update your calendar and repeat this process with each new assignment. Please see Figure 3–5 for an example of strategic planning with a large desk calendar.

Figure 3–5
Example of a large desk calendar.

Sunday	Monday	Tuesday	Wednesday	Thursday	Friday	Saturday
		1 Think of Possible Topics	2	3 Choose Paper Topic and Title	4	5 Library Research— 2.5 Hours
6 Library Research— 2.5 Hours	7 Mom's Birthday	8 Library Research— 2.5 Hours	9 Dance Class 4:00 p.m.	10	11 Library Research— 2.5 Hours	12 Develop Outline
13	14 Finish Outline	15	16	17 Write Rough Draft	18	19
20	21 Finish Rough Draft	22	23 Dance Class 4:00 p.m.	24 Rewrite Final Paper	25	26
27	28 Turn in Paper	29	30 Paper Due!!!			

September

The Daily To-Do List. Now you need to move on to a very important list, your daily to-do list. This should be done at your special study area with your calendar in front of you. A daily to-do list can be your most effective tool when referenced to your desk calendar. To construct this list, do the following:

1. Write down every activity, assignment, meeting, or promise that comes your way each day.
2. Do what activities you can as they occur, if time permits.
3. At the end of your day, prioritize your list. Place at top the tasks that need done the next day and mark them with an asterisk. Then list other tasks that would be nice to do and may even get you ahead. Remember to check your desk calendar for the next day when making this list. Now go to bed, secure in the knowledge that you do not have to worry about the next day.
4. Consult your list during the day, and cross off any task when completed. Crossing off the task should give you a sense of accomplishment. You should really derive pleasure from crossing off items on your list. This will reinforce your good behavior and keep you dedicated to your list. You should have all top-priority items crossed off at the end of the day.
5. Now make a new list for the next day. Get in the habit of spending a few minutes each day planning for the following day. It will help you greatly. This process will eventually become automatic.

Skill Application 3–6 Making a Daily To-Do List

a. Make a list of all tasks you want to accomplish tomorrow. Assign a priority by placing an asterisk or star next to the tasks that cannot be delayed and must be done tomorrow.

b. Place a number 1 by the tasks that are important and need to be done as soon as possible.

c. Place a number 2 next to the tasks that can be delayed for a while but, if time permits, could get you ahead of schedule. Limit yourself to only a few number 1 and 2 tasks.

d. Do this in consultation with your desk calendar for 7 consecutive days. Then evaluate your performance and learn how you can improve on your list-making skills and incorporate this process into your life.

Hint: Keep your lists as short and simple as possible—do not try to do everything in 1 day. Remember to cross off items when done. We purposely did not put a column for you to check off when each task is done. You can derive more pleasure and sense of accomplishment from crossing out the entire task.

Example

Things to Do Today List   Date: 11-5-23

Priority	Task
*	*Finish anatomy and physiology questions due Nov. 6.*
2	*Do library research for paper due Jan. 10.*

(continues)

(continued)

1	*Clean my room and organize my study area and closet.*
1	*Call the hospital to set up volunteer work for next week.*
*	*Get essential groceries for Grandma.*
*	*Soccer game at 1800.*
2	*Come up with an idea for science project, due Jan. 20.*
*	*Return Joshua's CPR manual, which he lent me last week.*

Your List

Things to Do Today List   Date: _____

Priority   **Task**

_____   _____
_____   _____
_____   _____
_____   _____
_____   _____
_____   _____

Things to Do Today List   Date: _____

Priority   **Task**

_____   _____
_____   _____
_____   _____
_____   _____
_____   _____
_____   _____
_____   _____

Things to Do Today List   Date: _____

Priority   **Task**

_____   _____
_____   _____
_____   _____

(continues)

(continued)

_____   _____

_____   _____

_____   _____

_____   _____

_____   _____

Things to Do Today List   Date: _____

Priority   **Task**

_____   _____

_____   _____

_____   _____

_____   _____

_____   _____

_____   _____

Capitalize on Peak Periods

During the study skills section, you assessed whether you were a morning or evening person. Most people are most productive in the morning, but we all differ. Know what times of day are most productive for you and schedule your more difficult tasks for these times.

You will also notice that your patients will also have peak periods when they respond to therapies better. In addition, they will have periods of distress, usually occurring at night. Have you ever noticed how you may feel sicker or more anxious at night?

Even seasonal changes can alter your productivity or feeling of well-being. Health studies show that depression and illness rise in areas where there is less sunlight. That is why a bright and cheery room in the dark of winter can be good medicine.

There are often low-value tasks that need done during the day. An example may be checking your e-mail. This low-value task needs to be completed several times during the day. Failure to do so may result in missing important information. Schedule this low-value task in between study sessions in order to break up the day.

Food **for** Thought 3–2

Peak Productive Periods

Why is it I get my best ideas during the morning while I'm shaving?

—Albert Einstein

When are you most productive?

_____

_____

Words to the Wise

You have done a great job planning. However, life rarely goes as planned. This is why you must be flexible and positive. If something unexpected comes up, do not panic or get negative and worry. This accomplishes nothing. Calm down, reorganize, and do what you can do.

Also know when you are overcommitted, and learn to say no. Remember, do not be rigid or fixated on your schedule or your lists. You do not have to make large lists. Make sure they are reasonable and give you time for yourself during the day.

Periodically reward yourself for getting all your tasks done. If you have a large task (e.g., that research paper), reward yourself along the way for each little step accomplished. This will help your motivation. But remember to save the biggest reward for when your large task is done. Here are some other things to "keep in mind."

1. Your goals can be changed.
2. Reward yourself when you reach short- and medium-range goals. This will reenergize you and give you a sense of movement and accomplishment toward your long-range goals.
3. You can make several more short- and medium-range goals. However, do not make more than one or two long-range goals per category or you may get overwhelmed.
4. Place your completed long-range goals in a prominent area in your portfolio and post a copy in your study area. This will keep them in your mind.

Congratulations, you now have good long-range goals established and one of the major tools (time management) to help you get there. Keep up the good work!

Summary

- Learning how to set proper goals will showcase your vision and direction in life. How many people do you know who say they are lost or have no direction in life? Many of them lack goals. But goals alone will not make everything all right. You need to know and practice the skills needed to obtain your goals.

- Setting goals and using good time management techniques are the tools you can use for your personal and professional success.

- Your goals should be Self-chosen, measurable, moderately challenging, attainable, and positive. They should include both personal and professional types of goals, should correspond with your personal brand, and should help to focus you on your journey toward professionalism.

- One major skill is effective time management. You may need to invest some time initially to learn these skills, but they will pay off in a big way. They will bring a sense of order and focus to your life. These skills will also help you free up time to enjoy yourself and recharge your energy.

- Time management techniques will help you to effectively and efficiently reach your goals. These techniques should include an assessment of time wasters in your life, using effective lists and capitalizing on your personal periods of peak productivity.

Case Study 3–1

Taisha had a difficult time in her Medical Assisting program and barely managed to graduate. She decided to try goal setting when she got hired in her first new job at a physician's office. She made only one goal, and it was as follows: "I want to be the office manager within a year." After her first year, Taisha was not the office manager and was very frustrated with her position and felt that goal setting was a bunch of "hogwash" and really doesn't work.

Did Taisha really understand the goal-setting process? What were the mistakes she made and how could she correct them?

_____

_____

_____

_____

Internet Activity   Using Internet search engines, try to find additional material on goal setting and time management that can help you and your fellow students. Some suggested keywords are goal setting, time management techniques, preventing procrastination, avoiding worry, and achieving goals. Write down something new that you found to share.

_____

_____

_____

_____

Chapter 4

Thinking and Reasoning Skills

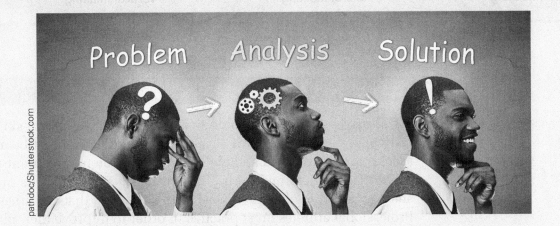

pathdoc/Shutterstock.com

Objectives

Upon completion of this chapter, you should be able to:

1. Differentiate the different types of thinking.

2. Differentiate between critical and creative thinking

3. Develop your creative and critical thinking skills.

4. Use an effective decision-making process to maximize your chances for success.

5. Begin to integrate critical and creative thinking skills into *your* life.

Key Terms

analogy	decision making	logical thinking
brainstorming	deductive reasoning	proactive thinking
cognitive processes	directed thinking	reactive thinking
creative thinking	inductive reasoning	undirected thinking
critical thinking	lateral thinking	vertical thinking

Introduction

We cannot solve our problems with the same thinking we used when we created them.

—Albert Einstein

Thinking is something we do every day. Good thinking skills are critical for a future health care professional. You must be able to assess, aid in diagnosis, develop and implement treatment plans. In addition, decision-making and problem-solving skills must be sharply honed to effectively deal with situations that can arise daily. Professional athletes must practice in order to improve their physical performances, and the same holds true for your mental performances. We can all become better thinkers with practice.

Have you ever "thought" about how you "think"? Psychologists, who specialize in studying how humans think, use the term **cognitive processes** to refer to the complex mental activities that compose thinking. These mental activities include using language, reasoning, solving problems, conceptualizing, remembering, imagining, and learning verbal material. These cognitive processes help us respond to our environment and greatly influence how we behave.

Several different types of "thinking" have been classified. These may include **logical**, **critical**, **creative**, **directed**, and **undirected thinking**. We discuss these thinking types individually and then relate how they can be integrated to make you an effective thinker. As an effective thinker, you will be able to maximize your decision-making and problem-solving skills. The development of these thinking skills will in turn make you an excellent health care professional.

Anticipatory Exercise 4–1 Thinking about Thinking

While the title of this exercise seems redundant, it really is a profound idea. Have you really ever thought about what type of thinker you are? Listed below are some thinking styles for you to consider before we get in to some "deep" thoughts on thinking.

(continues)

(continued)

Are you an optimistic or pessimistic thinker? Defend your answer.

_____

_____

_____

Are you a reactive or proactive thinker? Defend your answer.

_____

_____

_____

Are you a better creative or logical thinker or equally comfortable with both? Explain your preference.

_____

_____

Types of Thinking

We use logic several times each day. Any time we evaluate, judge, or decide something, we must rely on our logical thinking. Just what is logic? It is your ability to reason in a given situation. If you are cold, you will figure out a way to become warm. Your logic may tell you to get a coat, go inside, build a fire, or turn up the thermostat. You will choose what you think is the best response, given the situation and your previous knowledge. For example, if you did not know what a thermostat was, it could not be one of your options. So one part of logic relies on your past experience and knowledge. Another part of logical thinking relies on your ability to reason deductively and inductively.

Deductive reasoning is a form of logical thinking in which you reach a true conclusion based on true facts called premises. For example, you may have the following premises:

Premise: Patients with advanced lung disease will experience shortness of breath (SOB) on exertion.

Premise: Bob has advanced lung disease and is trying to help his daughter move.

Conclusion: Bob will experience SOB while helping his daughter move.

In this example, you used deductive reasoning to reach a true conclusion. The conclusion in deductive reasoning is always true if the premises are true. Because of your use of deductive reasoning, you can assist Bob by teaching him breathing retraining exercises and teaching him how and when to use his supplemental oxygen to breathe more effectively. This will decrease his SOB and make the moving day go a whole lot better.

In the previous example, you have just taken action that could prevent a potential crisis such as a cardiac arrest for Bob. This is called **proactive thinking**, or thinking ahead so that you are not in a crisis. Many people wait for the problem to occur and then react to the crisis. This is called **reactive thinking**. Which do you think is better?

Just For FUN 4-1

Mental Gymnastics

Use your deductive thinking skills to solve this problem:

A cat, a small dog, a goat, and a horse are named Angel, Beauty, King, and Rover. Using the clues that follow, find each animal's name.

Clue 1: King is smaller than both the dog and Rover.
Clue 2: The horse is younger than Angel and Beauty.
Clue 3: Beauty is the oldest and is a good friend of the dog.

Cat's name: _____   Goat's name: _____
Dog's name: _____   Horse's name: _____

Answers can be found in Appendix F.

Another type of logical thinking is **inductive reasoning**. Here you make your best guess based on the premises or facts. Your conclusion has a high probability of being true but is not always true. Here is an example of inductive reasoning:

Premise: People who smoke have an increased risk of getting lung cancer.

Premise: Maria smoked two packs of cigarettes for 20 years.

Conclusion: Maria will get lung cancer.

Although Maria's risk of getting lung cancer is much greater than that of someone who has not smoked and although it is possible that Maria may get lung cancer, the conclusion may not be true. She may never develop lung cancer. She may die from emphysema first or there may be several other possible outcomes. However, if she enters the emergency department with signs and symptoms that are consistent with cancer, your inductive reasoning, coupled with her past medical history, would lead you to suspect and test for the occurrence of lung cancer.

Skill Application 4–1 Logical Thinking

1. Define logical thinking in your own terms.

   _____

   _____

2. List three people you know personally whom you consider to be logical.

   _____

   _____

3. What is it about these individuals that led you to call them logical? List some personal attributes that you feel contribute to their logical thought process. Write a short paragraph for each individual to answer this question.

   _____

   _____

4. Interview at least one of these individuals and list three reasons why that person believes that they are a "logical person."

   a. _____

   b. _____

   c. _____

Critical and Creative Thinking

Much attention is being paid to developing critical thinking skills in students. However, there are many definitions and views on critical thinking, making this concept confusing. One definition of critical thinking is "the ability to suspend judgment, to consider alternatives, to analyze and evaluate." Another definition states "purposeful, goal-directed thinking," and there are still several other definitions. However, these definitions all include several thinking skills, such as the ability to develop a hypothesis, to test and rate possible solutions, and to maintain an objective viewpoint. Critical thinking skills relate to *analytical thinking*—the ability to objectively analyze a situation or set of facts. It should be noted that critical thinking skills (like all thinking skills) can be developed and improved on through practice.

Creative thinking also has several definitions and many misconceptions surrounding it. One common misconception is that creativity is only for artists, musicians, and writers. If we simply define creative thinking as "the generation of ideas that results in the improvement of the efficiency or the effectiveness of the system," we can see that it relates to all of us. We all want to "generate ideas and results that will not only improve the effectiveness of the health care system," but we can apply these same principles in improving our lives and those around to include our patients.

Psychologists who devote themselves to the study of the mind define creativity as the ability to see things in a new way and to help in problem solving. A worker who develops a better way to do the job, a parent who helps their child to learn a new skill or overcome a problem, and even someone who finds a better route on a map are all being creative. We use this skill every day of our lives without being fully aware of it.

Edward de Bono, an expert on thinking, coined the terms **vertical thinking** and **lateral thinking** to contrast critical and creative thinking. Vertical thinking relies on logic and each idea relates to the next. Vertical thinking allows us to make assumptions based on past experiences and relies on logical thinking, which includes deductive and inductive reasoning, which we have already discussed. Remember how we went in a stepwise fashion from premise to premise to conclusion?

Lateral thinking creates new ideas by making connections with no set pathway. Lateral thinking takes stored information and relates it in a previously unrelated manner. It generates the ideas that will later be evaluated by vertical, or logical, thinking modes. Some people think of this as "sideways thinking" because you are making connections with other thoughts versus the vertical step-by-step thinking. Figure 4–1 contrasts vertical and lateral thinking.

Figure 4–1
Contrasting vertical and lateral thinking.

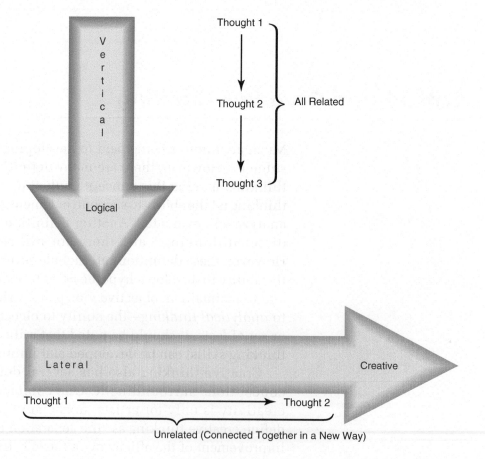

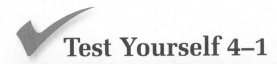

Test Yourself 4–1

Facts Concerning Creativity

True or False

1. _____ Intelligence is a key factor in creativity.

2. _____ The computer reduces our need to think for ourselves.

3. _____ Fear of failure blocks creativity.

Answers can be found in Appendix F.

Directed and Undirected Thinking

Most thinking is hard to categorize, and with all the terms, it can get quite confusing. One classification system simplifies thinking in terms of contrasting directed and undirected thinking. Both directed and undirected thinking involve some of the same mental processes such as memory, imagination, and association. Directed thinking is usually highly controllable, and a conscious effort is made to solve a specific problem or situation. The processes of learning, reasoning, and decision making are good examples of directed thinking.

Undirected thinking is looser and free flowing. Dreaming can be thought of as a type of undirected thinking process. This can include both daydreaming and dreaming while asleep. There is no apparent goal or specific problem, just a steady stream of thought. However, you will soon learn that this type of thinking can also assist in problem solving.

Just For FUN 4-2

Brain Teasers

1. If an electric train was traveling northwest on a railroad track in Greenland, in which direction would the smoke blow? _____

2. I have two coins and one is not a nickel. They total 55 cents. What are the two coins? _____

(continues)

(continued)

3. Count the number of squares in Figure 4–2. _____

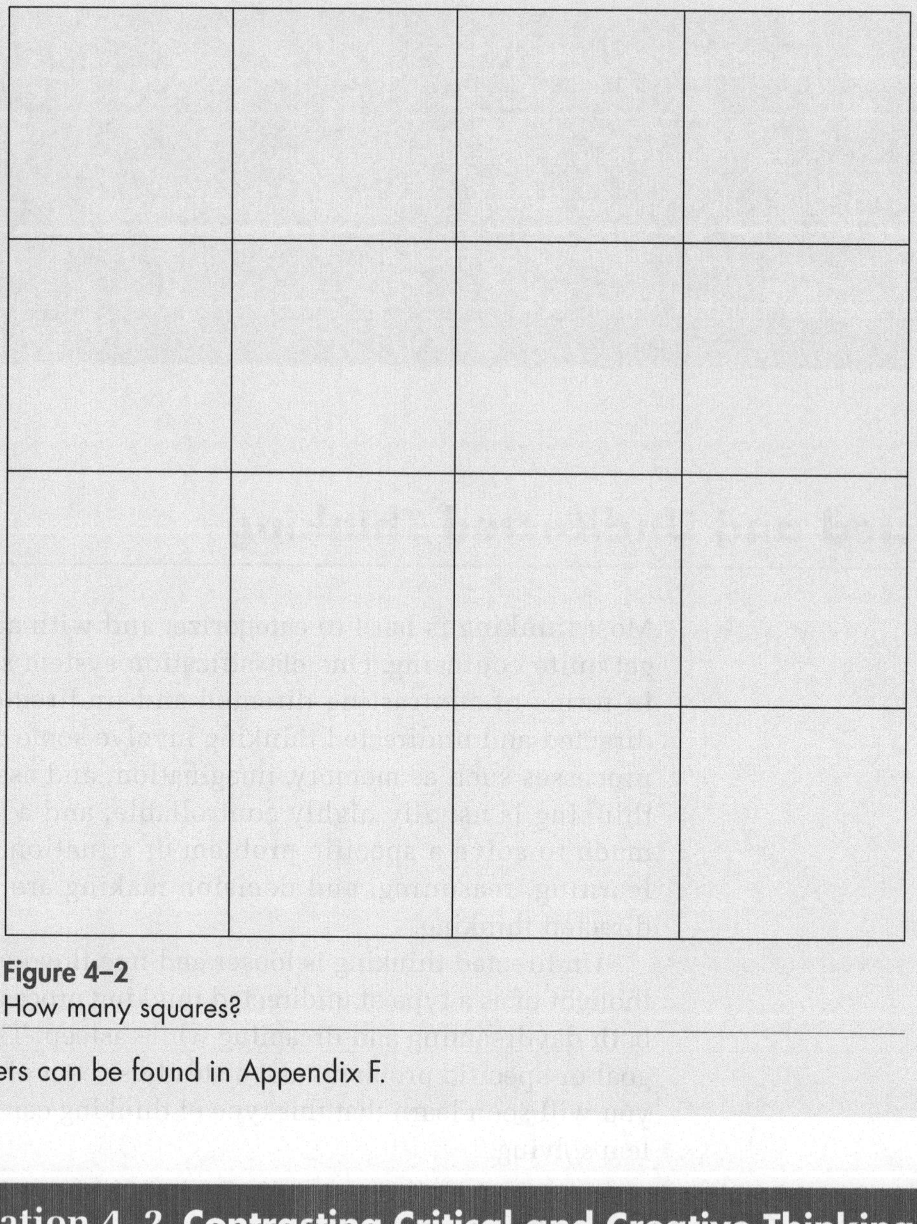

Figure 4–2
How many squares?

Answers can be found in Appendix F.

Skill Application 4–2 Contrasting Critical and Creative Thinking

In today's information age, everyone has access to a vast amount of knowledge. However, the successful people will be able not only to access this information but also to use their critical and creative thinking skills to develop breakthrough ideas and solutions. Research shows that critical and creative thinking skills can be taught and are key factors in personal and organizational excellence.

1. Define critical and creative thinking in your own words.

Critical thinking: _____

Creative thinking: _____

(continues)

(continued)

2. State whether you think the words listed below best reflect critical or creative thinking, or both.

Imagination: _____

Analytical: _____

Generative: _____

Selective: _____

Assessment: _____

Diagnosis: _____

Obtaining a medical history: _____

Evaluation: _____

Problem solving: _____

Brainstorming: _____

Daydreaming: _____

Prognosis _____

3. Circle any of the preceding words that are examples of directed thinking, and place a star by any examples of undirected thinking.

The Total Thinking Process

So far, we have talked about different types of thinking in definition and theory. Now let's move onto application of the thinking process.

Decisions

Decisions are something we make every day of our lives (Figure 4–3). Just what is **decision making**? Decision making is the act of making an informed choice between several alternatives to solve a problem or maximize an opportunity. Decision making helps you develop a definite course of action. Just look at some of the decisions you will make in a day.

Figure 4–3
When making decisions, it is important to consider the pros and cons of the choices available.

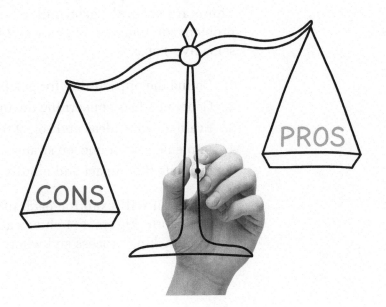

We must decide what time to get up, what clothes to wear, what we are going to do that day, what to eat, and so on. Many decisions have short-term effects and do not require a specific process. For example, you do not have to go through several steps in the decision-making process to decide what to eat. Usually, you look at the menu, decide what you like and how much you can spend, and then place your order. This is a short-term decision that will not have long-term effects, except maybe some nausea if the food was not prepared properly.

However, decisions that have long-term effects on our lives should have a specific process to maximize their successful outcome. For example, the following questions will all greatly influence your future:

What are my studying strategies?

What courses should I take to prepare for my career?

How do I maintain a healthy lifestyle?

Using the decision-making process will help you make more informed decisions that will lead to the results you desire. Decision making also helps *you* control the direction of your life instead of letting events or others take control of you. Decision making has some risks involved; however, it makes you confront your problems and take action that will minimize any risks.

The Decision-Making Process

The decision-making process can be called many things. Some refer to it as problem solving, but this makes it seem as if everything is a problem to be solved, which is not always the case. Sometimes you are looking at maximizing an opportunity, choosing the right path, creating a new opportunity, and yes, sometimes solving a problem. There are several variations of the decision-making process or problem solving, as some may call it, but they all have basically the same five steps:

1. Define the opportunity for positive change.
2. Generate ideas concerning the opportunity.
3. Evaluate your ideas and select the best one.
4. Implement your chosen strategy.
5. Evaluate the impact and modify accordingly.

Now you will examine each of these steps individually and in greater depth. Figure 4–4 shows a visualization of the steps in the decision-making process and where it will lead you.

Figure 4–4
The five steps in the decision-making process.

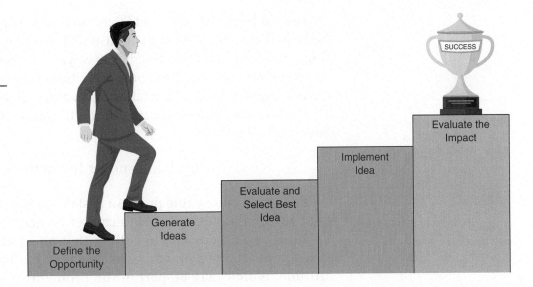

Step One: Define the Opportunity. Step one is to define the opportunity for positive change. Note that the first step does *not* say define the problem. This is because how you present this first step to your mind will greatly influence the outcome. So by looking at each major decision or problem as an opportunity for positive change, you are already on your way to a great solution.

Using this approach for the first step also increases proactive versus reactive thinking. Reactive thinking is when you wait for a problem to exist and then "react" and try to solve it. This is not very effective because now you may be dealing with a crisis situation that may be difficult to resolve. Proactive thinking is "looking ahead" and preventing problems from occurring. Now you can assess and optimize your environment with calm thinking and prevent many crisis situations from occurring.

You should be able to clearly state what the opportunity is in a manner that shows a positive outcome. Remember, how we state the problem greatly influences the rest of the process!

Here is a common "problem" stated in the sometimes hectic world of health care:

"I'm too busy."

The opportunity is not clearly stated, nor does it show any positive outcome. A problem stated in this manner is unlikely to be solved, and the person will only become more frustrated in time and always perceive themselves as too busy and take no action to solve this. However, this can be restated as follows:

"How do we streamline work habits to get the work done on time and allow professional development?"

Notice how this now presents an opportunity for professional development to occur when solutions are implemented to get the work done by streamlining work habits. You may find that there are several legitimate shortcuts that can be taken and not compromise high-quality care. This statement will force you to look at the way things are done and try to find better ways to do them. The reward will not be more work piled on, but rather time freed up for professional development, which is crucial in the health care professions.

Here is one more example of a complaint from nonphysician health care members:

"Physicians never listen to us."

Look how poorly this problem is stated. First, it implies that they are "never" listened to, which cannot be accurate. Second, using the term *never* leads you to believe that no solution exists. Do you suspect that the person who says this may not have a very positive attitude, which may be part of the problem? A better restatement would be as follows:

"How do we develop strategies to increase positive physician communication and interaction?"

This now clearly states what is hoped will be accomplished and what the positive outcomes will be. After having clearly stated the opportunity, you now need to gather all the pertinent data before going on to the next step, which will generate possible solutions. Get all the facts you can that relate to this opportunity. For example, if you were a supervisor and had a problem employee, your "opportunity" would be to achieve a positive change and have a happy productive employee. You would have to gather all the facts available as to why this employee is being unproductive before coming up with ideas. In summation, clearly state the opportunity with a positive outcome and gather all the "facts" together in step one. This step may take some time, but it will lay a solid foundation for success in your decision-making process.

Skill Application 4–3 Step One: Defining Your Opportunity for Positive Change

Pick one professional opportunity and one personal opportunity and state each in a positive manner. For example, the professional opportunity could be as follows: "How can I prepare myself to succeed in my chosen health career?" Notice that the opportunity is defined and stated in a positive manner. Even a personal problem can be stated in positive manner. For example, "How can I resolve the conflict with my coworker so that our work hours can be more enjoyable and productive?" Notice the positive opportunity. This is a lot better than, "Why is my coworker making my life miserable?" or "My coworker is impossible to work with!"

(continues)

(continued)

So now it is your turn to pick one professional and one personal opportunity to define. Give these careful thought because we will use these opportunities for the rest of this chapter in the decision-making process.

Professional opportunity: _____

Personal opportunity: _____

Are they clearly stated, and do they have positive outcomes?

_____

Now it is time to list all the pertinent facts concerning this opportunity. Try to steer clear of opinions. A fact is something that can be shown to be true. Opinions are beliefs based on values and assumptions and may or may not be true.

Now list all the facts that you can come up with concerning each potential opportunity. Spend some time on them and then take a break and get away. Allow the opportunity to ferment in your subconscious. Come back again and see if you can add to the lists.

Professional opportunity facts: _____

_____

Personal opportunity facts: _____

_____

Now you are ready to move on to the next step, where you will generate a host of ideas concerning your opportunity for positive change.

Step Two: Generate Ideas. Step two is to generate ideas concerning the opportunity. Now is the time to use your creative thinking skills and come up with ideas concerning the opportunity. It is important not to judge any of these ideas as good or bad. The key to this step is coming up with a quantity of ideas (Figure 4–5). Even what may seem to be far out ideas should be encouraged at this step.

How good are you at generating new ideas? If you consider yourself poor at this, you are not alone. Many people feel they are uncreative, but nothing could be farther from the truth. We are all creative, and there are ways we can enhance this creativity.

A lot of research was done concerning the left and right sides of our brain and creativity. It has been shown that the left side of our brain is more analytical, whereas the right side is more intuitive and creative. Some people have contended that creative individuals think mainly with the right side of the brain, whereas more logical or analytical thinkers are controlled by the left side of the brain. This was shown to be an oversimplification of what was occurring.

Figure 4–5
Engage your creative thinking skills when considering a new opportunity.

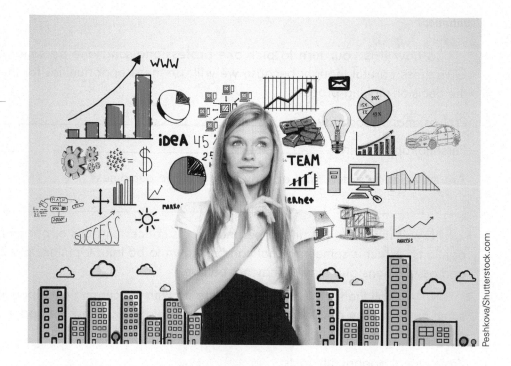

Peshkova/Shutterstock.com

During positron emission testing (which can measure and locate brain activity) of individuals performing creative tasks, the brain's electrical activity flickered between both hemispheres. This demonstrated the need, even in creative tasks, of connecting the right and left brain hemispheres. Therefore, it is important to make these cross-connections to enhance creative thinking. There are several techniques to enhance this.

Associative Thinking and Visualization. One method to force "cross-connections" is to sketch your opportunity or issue in the center of your paper. This is referred to as developing a concept map. Next, print key words and ideas and connect these to your central issue. Use colors and symbols to emphasize certain points. Study this visual picture and see if you can find new relationships, patterns, or ideas. It may take time, but the more ideas you develop, the better chance for a successful solution. Figure 4–6 is a visualization of a successful health career.

Brainstorming. Brainstorming is a powerful way to enhance creativity. This is when a small group of people (five to eight) collaborate and come up with ideas concerning an opportunity or issue that has been presented to them. However, it can be done with only two or more people. If done properly, it uses several brains that have different experiences, knowledge, and insights to greatly enhance the creative power. There are three important rules to make sure this process is effective.

Figure 4–6
Associative thinking and
visualization.

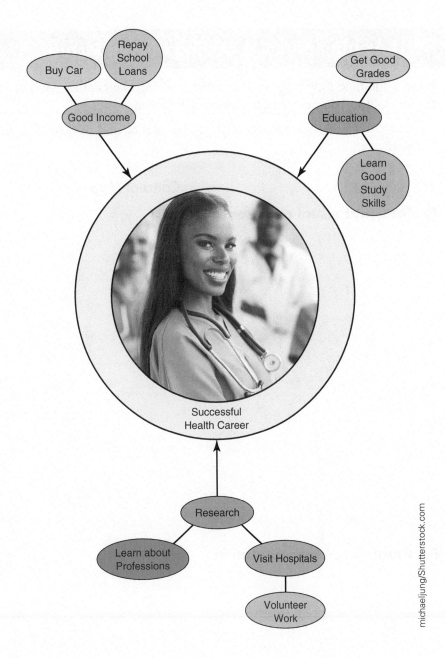

michaeljung/Shutterstock.com

Rule Number One: Withhold Premature Criticisms. Have you ever had someone be critical of an idea you gave in front of a group by saying something or using body language such as eye rolling? How did it make you feel? Did you want to give another idea?

Premature criticism will kill the creative process and should be avoided at all costs. Any idea, no matter how far-fetched, should be considered. Remember, the goal is not to come up with the best solution at this time. The goal here is to list all kinds of ideas that will be analyzed and evaluated in the next step. You might even combine some ideas at this stage.

Skill Application 4–4 Seeing the Big Picture

Now is the time to turn on your creative thinking. Remember, quantity of ideas is important at this stage; do not judge or evaluate ideas at this time.

Draw a visual representation of your personal and professional opportunity using associative thinking.

Concept Map

Professional visual representation

Personal visual representation

Rule Number Two: The Quantity of Ideas Is Important at This Stage, Not the Quality. The more ideas generated, the better the odds that a high-quality idea will emerge. Sometimes we are conditioned to believe that there is only one right answer and not being "right" means failure. This may be true in math, but in creative thinking, there are no "right" or "wrong" answers, only ideas.

Rule Number Three: Get Rid of Distractions. A nonthreatening atmosphere that is free of distractions provides the best environment for creative thinking. Distractions include noise, poor lighting, squeaky chairs, a telephone, pager, or a room that is either too hot or too cold.

Analogies. An **analogy** forces cross-connections between two unlike things. This can be helpful in generating ideas that would not have been thought of otherwise. Coors was paying millions of dollars to dispose of beer by-products, and creative consultants were brought in to come up with ideas. They used the analogy of Tom Sawyer, who convinced his friends that painting a fence was a privilege they should pay for. Coors employees used this analogy to come up with the idea to sell their beer by-products to the Japanese cattle industry. They now took something that was costly to dispose of and actually turned it into a profit much as Tom Sawyer convinced his friends it was a privilege to do his chore.

Many inventions came about as a result of analogies. Velcro was discovered because an inventor got a bunch of sticky burrs on his pants while walking through the woods. Analyzing the burrs, he developed Velcro, which has hundreds of uses. Using analogies can be both fun and creative in developing unique solutions.

Skill Application 4–5 Brainstorming Session

Following these guidelines, set up a brainstorming session to further develop ideas concerning your opportunities. If the personal opportunity is too sensitive to share, just do the professional one. However, you are encouraged to do both. Sharing ideas is a great way to enhance your personal growth as an individual. See Figure 4–7.

Guidelines for organizing a brainstorming session are as follows:

- Work in a group of at least three people and no more than eight.
- Choose a comfortable area that is well lighted and free of distractions.
- Assign one person to take notes and record ideas.
- Clearly state the opportunity and the facts concerning it.
- Be spontaneous and imaginative—do not judge or roll your eyes and encourage all to share.
- Listen to other people's ideas and build on them.
- Go for quantity of ideas.
- Do not evaluate someone else's idea.

(continues)

(continued)

1. List the ideas concerning your professional opportunity.

_____

_____

2. List the ideas concerning your personal opportunity.

_____

_____

3. Jot down some of your impressions of the brainstorming session. What did you dislike?

_____

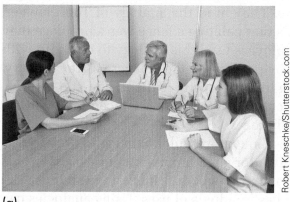

(a)   (b)

Robert Kneschke/Shutterstock.com

Figure 4–7
Which brainstorming session is more effective?

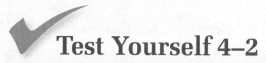

Test Yourself 4–2

Barriers to the Creative Process

Place a check beside any of the barriers to the creative process you may have.

1. _____ Fear of losing control: Are you threatened by allowing others to give ideas because you feel you may not be "in charge"?

2. _____ Resistance to change: When change is proposed, do you feel "this is the way it always has been done, why should we look for a better way?"

3. _____ Premature criticism: Do you immediately judge someone else's idea as good or bad?

4. _____ "Borrowing of ideas": Do you take credit for others' ideas? Do you think people would give additional ideas to a person who they think will take the credit?

5. _____ Procedural dependency: Do you think that there must be only one right way to do something?

Tapping into Your Subconscious. The subconscious is a powerful ally in generating ideas about a problem or situation. The subconscious protects us and helps us survive without our even knowing that it is working. It is the part of our mind working just underneath the surface which is what "sub" means. This is why many people will have a solution to a problem appear as if by magic when they were not consciously thinking about it. Letting go of a problem allows it to stew in the subconscious, where new ideas and relationships can be established. Simply slowing your mind if it is going a million miles per hour down allows your subconscious to bubble up and also allows you to think more clearly. This activity may seem simple. Try to think about *absolutely nothing* for 1 minute. Can you do it? It is not as easy as it sounds.

> Often, when the conscious forcing of the problem to solution has failed, the incubational process succeeds.
>
> —Eugene Raudsepp, Pres., Princeton Creative Research

Skill Application 4–6 Letting Go and Capitalizing on Peak Periods of Creativity

Choose some type of activity you enjoy. It could be reading, playing a sport, walking in the woods, and so on. Right before you engage in the activity, clearly state your opportunity. Take a couple of slow, deep breaths while visualizing it in your mind. Now do your activity and forget the problem. Immerse yourself in your activity. See if in the next day or two an idea comes to you when you "think" you were not "thinking" about the problem. Careful, you may even dream about it. Write down any ideas that came to you.

_____

_____

Capitalizing on Peak Creativity

We all have times when we are more creative. For example, some people are most creative on their morning drive to work. They capitalize on this by being ready to record any good ideas that come to them.

1. When are you most creative? _____

2. In what environment are you most creative? _____

3. How do you capitalize on your peak periods of creativity? _____

Step Three: Evaluate and Select the Best Idea. Step three is to evaluate your ideas and select the best one. In this step, you shift to your logical or analytical thinking to evaluate each idea or combination of ideas for its successful outcomes. Basically, you are weighing the pros and cons of each idea in order to choose the best idea that will give you your desired outcome.

You now need to select or choose from among the various ideas, the course of action that will provide the greatest chance for success. You can visually test each of them by imagining that each has already been put into effect. Consider the short- and long-term effects of each idea. Evaluate their merit and then make your choice.

Skill Application 4–7 Step Three of the Decision-Making Process: Evaluate and Select the Best Idea

Now you must evaluate and choose the ideas that are best suited to achieve a positive outcome. For the following exercises, refer to the ideas generated in the previous exercise.

For each idea generated, spend some time visualizing, imagining, and even daydreaming what would happen if you chose and implemented it. After you do this for each idea, list any short- and long-term positive or negative outcomes.

Professional Opportunity

Idea 1:

Short-term positive outcomes: _____

Short-term negative outcomes: _____

Long-term positive outcomes: _____

Long-term negative outcomes: _____

Idea 2:

Short-term positive outcomes: _____

Short-term negative outcomes: _____

Long-term positive outcomes: _____

Long-term negative outcomes: _____

Idea 3:

Short-term positive outcomes: _____

Short-term negative outcomes: _____

Long-term positive outcomes: _____

Long-term negative outcomes: _____

Personal Opportunity

Idea 1:

Short-term positive outcomes: _____

Short-term negative outcomes: _____

(continues)

(continued)

Long-term positive outcomes: _____

Long-term negative outcomes: _____

Idea 2:

Short-term positive outcomes: _____

Short-term negative outcomes: _____

Long-term positive outcomes: _____

Long-term negative outcomes: _____

Idea 3:

Short-term positive outcomes: _____

Short-term negative outcomes: _____

Long-term positive outcomes: _____

Long-term negative outcomes: _____

Step Four: Implement the Idea. Step four is to implement your chosen strategy. This is when you put your idea into action. Here, you must ask several questions: What is the best way to implement your chosen solution? What factors may have to be considered in this implementation process? How do you need to communicate this idea and to whom? Once it is implemented, you can proceed to step five. Do the skill application that will walk you through this step.

Skill Application 4–8 Step Four: Implementation

If you have more ideas, evaluate them using this same system. Now choose either a personal or professional idea or ideas you think should be implemented and write it here.

_____

_____

_____

_____

Take at least a few days away from this activity, and then come back and review your work. If you still think you have come up with the best possible solution, move on to the last activity.

(continues)

(continued)

Answer the following questions before implementing your solutions.

1. Will implementing this idea have an impact on others? If so, list those people and what type of impact it may have. _____

2. What is the best way to communicate this idea to all concerned? _____

3. When is the best time to implement this idea? _____

4. What are the best steps in implementing this solution? _____

Step Five: Evaluate Impact. Step five is to evaluate the impact of your idea and modify it accordingly. Does your chosen idea create the positive opportunity or solve the problem? Is the outcome desirable? If the solution is not desirable, consider another one, rethink all possible solutions, or reevaluate the problem. Get feedback from as many sources as possible to determine whether your idea is having a positive impact. The more feedback you receive, the better your ability to evaluate and modify the outcomes.

The five steps to the decision-making process may seem like a lot to go through, but it is well worth the effort. With practice, these steps will become second nature and will be used almost effortlessly. Besides, you are worth the best effort when making the truly important decisions, which will have a major impact on your life.

Skill Application 4–9 Step Five of the Decision-Making Process: Evaluation

Now implement the solution. After an appropriate period, evaluate its impact and modify it accordingly. Your answers to the following questions will assist you.

1. What positive outcomes should I begin to see? _____

2. When should I see these outcomes? _____

3. Who can give me appropriate feedback? _____

4. How will I know that the solution is working? Be as specific as possible.

_____

Do not be afraid to modify your solution when you obtain your feedback. This is normal and occurs often.

Summary

- Thinking is something you do every day of your life. Understanding the various types of thinking will make you better able to analyze a situation and develop an effective idea or solution.

- The decision-making process combines the various types of thinking into an effective strategy for problem solving. The five steps to the decision-making process are as follows:

  1. Define the opportunity for positive change.
  2. Generate ideas concerning the opportunity.
  3. Evaluate your ideas and select the best one.
  4. Implement your chosen strategy.
  5. Evaluate the impact and modify your idea accordingly.

- Learning about and practicing these steps will make you an excellent decision maker.

- You can enhance your creative thinking by using associative thinking, visualization, brainstorming, the use of analogies, and tapping into the power of your subconscious.

Just For FUN 4–3

Mental Flexibility

This is an interesting test of your mental flexibility and creativity. Many people report that the answers come to them after they put the test aside. This concept is discussed in the section on creative thinking in problem solving. For now, just have fun and see how many answers you can get.

Instructions: Each equation contains initials of words that will make it correct. For example, "7 = N. of D. in a W." would be 7 = *number of days in a week*. Now try the rest.

26 = L. of the A.: _____

12 = S. of the Z.: _____

52 = C. in a D. (without the Js): _____

 8 = P. in the S. S.: _____

88 = P. K.: _____

18 = H. on a G. C.: _____

29 = D. in F. in a L. Y.: _____

206 B. in the B.: _____

 4 = Q. in a G.: _____

 2 = P. in a Q.: _____

 8 = S. on a S. S.: _____

See if you can come up with five on your own to share with your classmates.

Answers can be found in Appendix F.

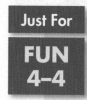

Just For FUN 4–4

Do Not Be Afraid to Color Outside of the Lines

Connect all the nine dots in Figure 4–8 with four straight lines without lifting your pencil from the paper.

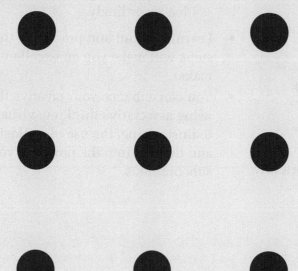

Figure 4–8
Can you solve this?

Here is a hint:

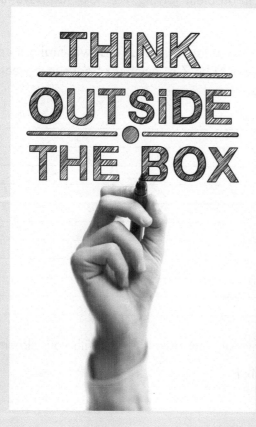

Peshkova/Shutterstock.com

Answers can be found in Appendix F.

Case Study 4–1

A health care department has decided to implement brainstorming as a method to increase ideas from the employees that can improve communication and morale. During the first brainstorming session, no one was sure exactly what the session was about and there were many distractions of noise and people moving about. During the early part of the session, the supervisor rolled her eyes and let out a heavy sigh when an employee offered up an idea. Very few ideas were generated and little interaction then took place.

Do you think this was a properly run brainstorming session? What do you think actually happened to morale and communication?

_____

_____

Why were there few or no ideas and little interaction during this session?

_____

_____

What could be done to improve the session and make it a positive and productive experience for all?

_____

_____

Case Study 4–2

This case is all about putting what you learned in this chapter to action. Working in a small group of at least two people, select one of the ideas below or come up with one of your own.

- Develop a health care career exploration fair that will help your fellow students.
- Develop a health care community experience that will help your community.

Write down your chosen opportunity for positive change:

_____

_____

Now go through the brainstorming process with your group and generate ideas around your chosen opportunity.

_____

_____

_____

_____

Evaluate and select the best idea.

_____

_____

_____

Describe how you will implement your idea.

_____

_____

_____

Remember, if you follow through on your opportunity for positive change, evaluate the impact!

Internet Activity

Using Internet search engines, find additional material on thinking and reasoning skills that can help you and your fellow students. Some suggested keywords are creative thinking, critical thinking, problem solving, reasoning skills, lateral thinking, and decision making. Write down something new that you found to share.

Chapter 5
Stress Management

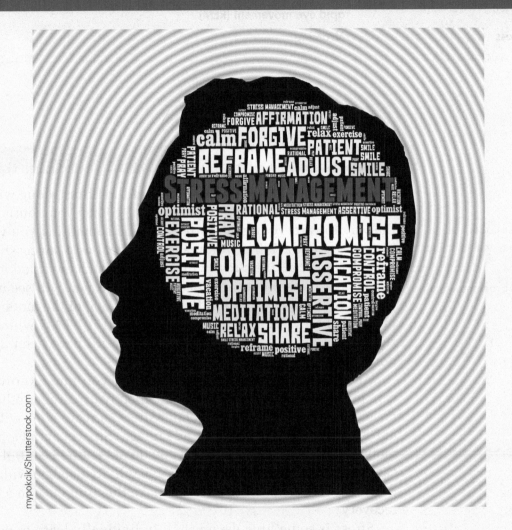

mypokcik/Shutterstock.com

Objectives

Upon completion of this chapter, you should be able to:

1. Define stress.

2. Contrast "good" and "bad" stress.

3. Identify your personal stress signals.

4. Identify the different types of stress and their effects on your mind and body.

5. Develop personalized social, physical, and emotional coping techniques to deal with stress.

Key Terms

bad stress	meditation	sadness
constructive concern	multicompetencies	STAT
depression	multiskilling	stress reaction
distress	nonrapid eye movement	worry
eustress	rapid eye movement (REM)	
good stress	reframing	

Introduction

Most folks are about as happy as they make up their minds to be.

—Abraham Lincoln

You now have your goals and vision of the future along with effective time management techniques to help you on your journey. Along the way toward your goals, stress will be something you will have to contend with. When you reach your goal as a successful health care professional, the stress will not end. Watch any good television show or read any novel about a hospital and you will see many situations that can be stressful. For example, one of the more common medical abbreviations used in the hospital is **STAT**, which means right away, or as we jokingly say, you should have been there and done it by now.

As a future health care professional, you must know how to care for yourself first before you can effectively care for others. This means that you need to learn about stress, how to cope with stress, and how to use stress to your advantage. Stress can be a powerful motivator for growth. However, if you do not learn to control it, stress can control your life and take a terrible toll. Remember, without you, there will not be someone there to make the difference in a patient's recovery.

Stress is something we must all individually learn to deal with. Many people do not realize that stress can be used as a positive force if managed correctly. This chapter and its related activities will help you learn how to cope with and harness your stress in a positive way. The health care environment will certainly give you much practice in dealing with stress. Besides, if you cannot handle stress, what kind of message does that send to your patient?

Anticipatory Exercise 5–1   **Stress in Health Care**

What types of stress do you think you will encounter as a health care professional? What about dealing with patients or their families?

How will you handle your first patient's death?

What if you make a mistake in treating a patient?

What if you entered the wrong medical code for a procedure and the patient's insurance won't cover it and the medical office does not get paid?

These questions should cause you to think and probably will cause some stress. Feeling some stress is good and normal. Stress can help you grow and prepare for what lies ahead. The good news is that you can learn to use stress to your advantage. Learning how to deal with stress will allow you to have a much fuller and more rewarding life. Making stress your friend will prepare you for the wonderful challenges life has to offer.

Understanding Stress

This chapter discusses the different types of stress. Most notably and to keep it relatable, you can have good stress that gets you "up" and makes you sharp for the task at hand. You can also have bad stress that inhibits your ability to do well.

The key point is how you perceive the stress and whether you control it, or it controls you. Let us begin by exploring the types of stress in your life.

To be able to conquer and harness stress to your advantage, you must first understand what stress is all about. It is important to realize that no situation or event by itself causes us stress. Rather it is how we "perceive" a situation that causes stress. It is our internal response to external stimuli.

For example, two individuals may receive an injection. They will both undergo the *same* procedure with the *same* technician in the *same* environment. You would think their reaction should also be the *same*. However, one individual may not feel any stress or anxiety at all, whereas the other may be highly stressed at the thought of getting a shot. Therefore, stress, like beauty, is in the eye of the beholder. Stress occurs as a result of how we interpret and react to a situation or event, as in Figure 5–1. It can be positive or negative, major or minor.

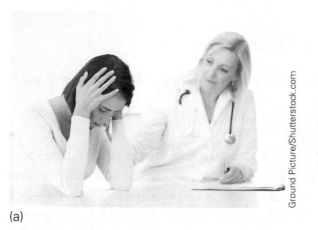

(a)

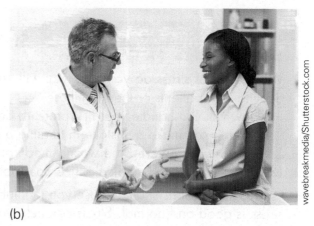

(b)

Figure 5–1
These patients are both interacting with a health care provider yet are experiencing different reactions.
Who perceives stress?

Just For

FUN 5–1

Expressing Your Stress

There are many common expressions that relate to stress. Some examples include the following:

- I was so scared I lost my breath.
- I was breathless with excitement. (Remember stress can be good.)
- I can now breathe easier.
- My heart was pounding.
- My brain is fried.
- My stomach was twisted in knots.

Notice how these relate stress to physiologic activities. The mind and body are truly related. What implications can this have for your patients? Can you think of other statements?

Stress can have many definitions. For now, we will define the **stress reaction** as "how our mind and body react to an environment that is largely shaped by our perceptions of an event or situation." Now that we have defined the stress reaction, let us take a closer look at the different types of stress and the physical and psychological reactions that can occur.

Types of Stress and Its Effects

The first time you are called on to perform cardiopulmonary resuscitation (CPR) on someone whose heart has stopped beating is probably going to be a stressful event in your life. Even though you practiced and trained hard, you are still uncertain of how it will be in a real

life-and-death situation. This is normal. Your physical and psychological symptoms may include the following:

- Increased adrenaline levels for more energy
- Faster heart rate (tachycardia) to supply more oxygen to muscles
- Increased blood pressure to get more blood flow to the brain
- Pupil dilation to bring in more light
- Faster breathing (tachypnea) to bring in more oxygen
- Heightened state of awareness to focus on the job at hand
- Mild level of anxiety to keep you sharp and not take the situation too lightly

These can all be helpful reactions that enhance your performance. Therefore, you can have **good stress** and **bad stress**. The key again is balance or moderation. Figure 5–2 graphically illustrates good versus bad stress. A little stress will get you "up" for the task at hand. However, if you let stress get out of hand and panic, you now have bad stress and your anxiety level rises to the point where you perform poorly or even not at all.

Figure 5–2
Good stress and
bad stress.

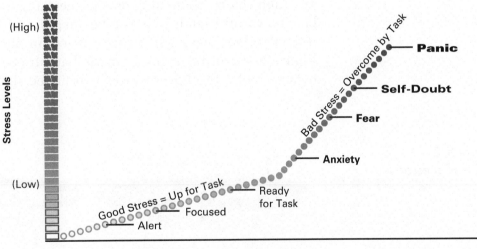

Food for Thought 5-1

Technical Terms

Hans Seyle, the father of stress research, coined the term **eustress** to describe positive stress. "Eu" means good or well. Seyle used the term **distress** for negative stress. This worktext will simply use the terms *good* and *bad stress* to help personalize the terms in your life.

Both positive and negative experiences can cause stress. For example, if your first CPR experience was successful, it will cause less stress than a negative experience. The mere fact that this is your "first" real CPR experience makes it stressful because the experience is unpredictable or unknown. Afterward, you will have gained experience. Even if you made mistakes, you will learn from those mistakes and know what to expect the next time. Therefore, unpredictable events are more stressful than predictable events.

Stress can also relate to time. We all have temporary stressors (factors that cause stress) in our lives. However, when a stressor becomes constant, it has serious effects on our body and mind. Continual or constant bad stress can lead to the following:

- High blood pressure, heart attack, or stroke
- Lack of mental focus
- Lack of sleep or insomnia
- Decreased immune system functioning
- Depression and personality changes

Temporary controlled stress can help us perform better. Indeed, any time you try something new or meet a new challenge, stress can be a powerful friend. This is how we grow and develop. Continual uncontrolled stress will exact a price on our minds and bodies. Figure 5–3 contrasts good versus bad stress. Trying to maintain balance and control over stress is discussed shortly.

Figure 5–3
Types of stressors.

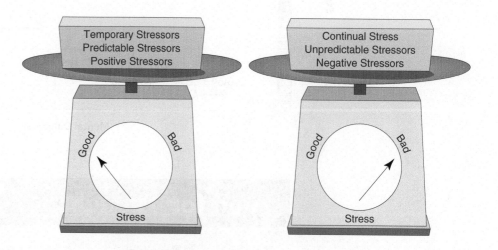

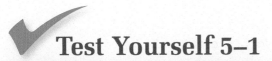

Test Yourself 5–1

Do You Need This Chapter?

Rate the following statements with numbers 1 through 4 as follows:

1. Rarely   2. Sometimes   3. Often   4. Mostly

1. _____ I feel tired.
2. _____ I worry a lot about problems or how things are going to turn out.
3. _____ I can spot all the things others are doing wrong.
4. _____ I need to be perfect at what I do.
5. _____ I skip my exercise sessions.
6. _____ I feel sad.
7. _____ I am very competitive and need to win to feel good about myself.
8. _____ I take on everyone else's problems.
9. _____ I try to control others.
10. _____ I cannot do anything right.
11. _____ I avoid risks for fear of failure.
12. _____ I let my work pile up.
13. _____ I feel like I am being pulled in all directions.
14. _____ I have a very negative attitude.
15. _____ I get headaches.
16. _____ I have too much to do and too little time to do it.
17. _____ I overreact to situations.
18. _____ I feel guilty if I relax and do nothing.
19. _____ I talk very quickly.
20. _____ I get angry easily.

Total Points _____

Now use your total to see where you stand:

Over 60–80   This chapter could be a life-changing experience.

50–59   You desperately need to work on this chapter.

40–49   You would gain moderate benefit from this chapter.

30–39   You are doing pretty good but can improve slightly.

20–29   Maybe you should write a book on handling stress.

Skill Application 5–1 Questions about Stress

1. Identify three situations where stress was a positive experience for you.

    a. _____

    b. _____

    c. _____

(continues)

(continued)

2. Why do people who think negatively experience a lot of stress?

_____

3. How do you know when you are getting stressed out?

_____

4. List five physical or emotional signs you have when experiencing negative stress.

   a. _____

   b. _____

   c. _____

   d. _____

   e. _____

A Simplified Stress Management System

There are several systems of stress management. We believe the simplest and most logical is to break down stress management into the following three areas:

- Recognize your stress signals and stress producers.
- Be concerned but try to avoid worrying!
- Develop positive coping strategies.

First, recognizing your own stressors and the symptoms they cause can help you determine when your stress is out of balance. These signals can be valuable to your good health and positive attitude. They represent a "wake-up call" that says you need to cope with what is going on in your life before it overtakes you.

Second, try to minimize **worry** in your life. While we all worry, worry is wasted negative energy. If you can learn to minimize worrying (and you can), you will gain back energy to grow. We will work more on "how to do this" shortly.

Finally, part of the stress management system is developing effective positive coping mechanisms to deal with and minimize the negative stressors in your life. These are not only very effective but also very fun if approached with a positive attitude. See Figure 5–4.

Recognizing Your Stress Signals

As already stated, a certain amount of stress is normal. We need it to develop and grow. However, going beyond minimal stress levels for sustained periods can be harmful. You need to determine when you are losing balance. The best way is to look for signs or indicators that the stress is too much. Table 5–1 shows the physical changes and emotional changes that signal too much stress.

Figure 5–4
Three-point stress management system.

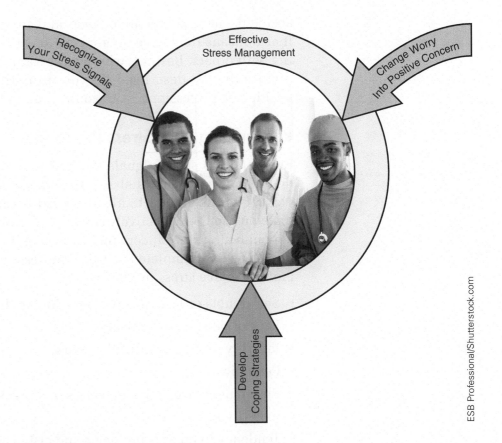

Table 5–1
The Physical and Emotional Signs of Stress

Physical Changes	Emotional Changes
Headaches	Lack of concentration
Shortness of breath	Irritability
Increased pulse rate	Anger
Nausea	Mood swings
Insomnia	Over reactiveness
Fatigue	Depression
Neck or back pain	Eating disorders
Dermatological problems	Anxiety
Chronic constipation/diarrhea	Low self-image
Nervous habits	Hopeless feelings

It is important to differentiate **depression** from **sadness.** If someone is sad after a painful disappointment or the loss of a loved one, this is a normal part of the grieving process. However, if the sadness remains for a prolonged period and interferes with the ability to go about your daily business, it becomes depression. Again, moderation is the key.

Looking at the list of stress signs in Table 5–1 should paint a pretty good visual picture of what high levels of stress can cause. It is no wonder that individuals who cannot handle stress have more accidents, have poorer attendance, and are unable to study and learn. It also means they have poorer relationships and difficulty interacting with others. Besides, who would want to constantly feel like the picture the list describes? Do you think this would be the kind of health care professional you would want to treat you?

Recognizing Your Stress Producers

Everyone has stress signals that tell them when they need to slow down and reevaluate their stress management. When these signals occur, sit back and try to identify what is causing this extra stress so that you can then effectively cope. The following list represents some common stress producers that can quickly get out of hand. This by no means is a complete list, but it represents some of the more common excessive stress producers:

- Self-doubts or lack of confidence in our abilities
- Lack of personal organization
- Inability to plan or prioritize work
- Perfectionism
- Placement of excessive demands on ourselves
- Inability to say no
- Tendency to take all problems and criticisms personally
- Inflexibility and lack of openness to change

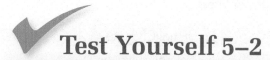 **Test Yourself 5–2**

How Many Stress Signals Do You Have?

How many of the following signals do you have on a regular basis (once or twice every week)? If you checked two or fewer signals, you are doing pretty good and need minor improvement. If you checked three or more, you need to work hard on how you are handling stress.

1. _____ Headaches
2. _____ Shortness of breath
3. _____ Fast or irregular pulse
4. _____ Nausea
5. _____ Insomnia
6. _____ Difficulty eating
7. _____ Sadness
8. _____ Chronic fatigue
9. _____ Irritability
10. _____ Hostility
11. _____ Mood swings
12. _____ Feelings of being overwhelmed
13. _____ Difficulty concentrating
14. _____ Neck or back pain
15. _____ Chronic diarrhea

Finally, negative thinking or thought patterns can add excessive stress to our lives. People who are in the habit of thinking in negative ways feel out of control. They have thoughts such as "I'll never learn this technique" or "My patients will never like me." All these thoughts are sending a message that "You are helpless and 'never' will accomplish your goal." You have already set up a negative self-fulfilling prophecy. The computer programmers have a saying "GIGO," which stands for garbage in, garbage out. Do you see how this can relate to negative thinking or programming?

Skill Application 5–2 Sources of Stress

This chapter describes a three-point system for stress management. We will now work on the first point, which is recognizing your stress signals and producers.

Your stress signals are your early warning detection system that says you have to do something. That something will come soon. For now, learn to identify the sources of stress in your life and recognize the signals when stress is out of control.

Stress can come from several different sources. For example, it can come from your personal life, work, or school. Identify two major sources that produce stress in your personal life and two sources of stress in school.

1. Personal stressor 1: _____

2. Personal stressor 2: _____

3. School stressor 1: _____

4. School stressor 2: _____

Skill Application 5–3 Your Physical Signs of Stress

For each personal and school stressor, list three physical/mental symptoms you experience when the stress gets excessive.

1. Personal stressor 1: _____

2. Personal stressor 2: _____

3. School stressor 1: _____

4. School stressor 2: _____

Change Worry into Positive Concern

Before developing specific coping strategies, special mention needs to be given to worry. Worry is destructive and wasteful energy. If we can learn to minimize worrying, we will gain that energy back to do something about what we were worrying about in the first place.

Convert your useless worrying to positive **constructive concern**. Being concerned means that you may ask yourself what you can do to improve the situation and then calmly proceed to do it. Being concerned means that you do not engage in self-pity or exhaust your energy mulling over the past. You live in the present and learn to take appropriate action when needed.

Again, the difference between worry and concern is a matter of degree and most importantly action. It is important to be concerned about people and issues. If we let our concerns get out of control to the point of rendering us ineffective, it becomes worrying.

Food for Thought 5–2

Classic Wisdom

I'm an old man and have known a great many problems, most of which never happened to me.

—Mark Twain

What was Mark Twain trying to tell us?

_____

_____

_____

_____

Skill Application 5–4 Turning Worry into Positive Concern

Now we move on to the second point of the three-point system. Turing worries into positive concern! Although a very short section was devoted to "worrying" in this chapter, it is one of the most destructive activities we can engage in. Worrying does nothing but wear us down both physically and mentally. However, being concerned means that we calmly analyze the situation and do what is needed to be done to improve it.

1. Write down the one thing you worry the most about. Be specific. Remember, worry is when "it kind of drives you crazy thinking about it."

2. Now write down what you can do about it. In other words, what steps can be taken to improve the situation? Again, be specific.

3. Now write down what *you are* going to do about it. Your answer should be pretty much the same as that for the previous question. Do you get the point we are emphasizing?

4. Finally, write down when you are going to start doing it!

_____

Notice there is not much room for your response to number 4. This emphasizes the point to *do* something about your worrying and to do it *now*. Appropriate and timely action will make your life a lot more fun and productive. It will also slow down that constant mind talk we all do, which speeds up a zillion times when we worry.

Effective Coping Strategies

Remember that the most important aspect of stress is that it is individually determined. Its meaning lies within us. Therefore, we are the ones to determine what is stressful and whether we are going to use stress to our advantage or let it use us. It should logically follow, if *we* determine the level of stress, *we* should be able to control it.

Someone once said that you do not get ulcers from what you eat, but rather from what is eating you. It is important to cope with stress before you suffer from stress overload or burnout. There are two basic ways you can cope with stress. The first is to effectively cope with the emotional side of stress. The second is to deal with its physical side. Stress can wreak havoc on our emotional well-being. However, we can use our minds to control stress and make it a positive influence. The five main strategies to emotionally handle stress include:

- Recognizing and eliminating stressors
- Reframing your thinking
- Using good time management
- Developing a social support group
- Rejuvenating yourself

Recognize and Eliminate Stressors. First, it is important to know what personally stresses *you* out and when you are getting out of control. One simple yet effective method is to write down your stressors. Now think of ways you can regain control over or eliminate the stress completely. However, realize there are some stressors that you can do something about and some that you cannot.

For example, you will eventually be faced with treating a terminally ill patient. A terminal illness is untreatable and irreversible. This certainly causes stress for your patient. The patient may be difficult to deal with but think of what they are going through. This situation can cause stress for you. You cannot change the stress caused by knowing that your patient is going to die. However, you can make a big difference in how your patient dies. Your care and support can increase your patient's quality of life during the remaining time and allow them to put personal affairs in order. You can make it the best death possible. Your concern and subsequent actions can truly make a difference.

Reframe Your Thinking. You can also cope with stress by changing how you think about a stressful situation. By **reframing** your perceptions, you can change the meaning of an event. Reframing means to rename in a positive sense. The Chinese word for problem means opportunity. If we can learn to look at what we perceive to be problems as actually opportunities, our stress would reduce drastically.

For example, **multiskilling** and **multicompetencies** are two important concepts in health care. This means you may be cross-trained to do other basic jobs. Most allied health professionals are being trained to perform vital sign assessment and basic patient care (e.g., bathing, turning) to assist nursing personnel in units where they may be stationed. As an occupational therapist, this may cause stress because you think it is "not your job" or you are anxious about performing certain skills. However, an excellent occupational therapist would understand the necessity and reframe their thinking as follows: "This will give me an opportunity to learn new skills that I can add to my résumé. In addition, it will make me more valuable to my organization and increase my job security. Besides, it will be fun to work more hand in hand with the nurses in basic patient care."

Use Good Time Management. You must master the effective time management techniques discussed in Chapter 3 to reduce stress. Especially, remember to say "no" to additional projects, responsibilities, or demands when accepting them would mean being overcommitted. Note that complaining is not the same as saying no. Complaining does not relieve stress, it reinforces it. By being organized and not allowing your work to pile up, you will greatly reduce the stress in your life.

Develop a Social Support Group. Your family, friends, and teachers can provide support in dealing with stress. Research suggests that emotional support helps people deal with stress. That is why it is so important to develop a social network and spend time with family and friends each week. Even if these are just people you trust to listen to you, this will allow you to vent some of your stress. Their outside objective perceptions may also help the situation. In other words, they may see things you cannot because you are too emotional about the situation.

As a health care professional you become an integral part of the patients' support systems. They rely on your medical expertise to assess and treat their condition. They also rely on your emotional support to help them through their stressful periods.

Rejuvenate Yourself. Learn to rejuvenate or recharge yourself when stress gets the best of you. You can do this in many ways. For example, take a break from your routine and do enjoyable activities or hobbies. Take a mental health vacation (a day or half a day to yourself) or, if you can, a real minivacation. Remember, vacation means to vacate and get away. Do you know people who take vacations and try to cram everything into a point where they need a vacation after their vacation?

Listening to your favorite music can also help. Research has proven music affects many of the major systems of our body. Music can both stimulate and relax you, depending on the type. It is best to listen to soothing music during periods of excessive stress.

Finally, do not forget to have a good laugh. The average 4-year-old child laughs every few minutes. Laughter helps bring you back in perspective, and besides it feels good. Laughter also helps you physically by lowering blood pressure, releasing endorphins, and stimulating the pleasure centers of the brain. You will notice that patients with a good sense of humor are more compliant and respond better to treatment.

Have you ever said to someone, "Someday we'll look back on this and laugh?" Chances are it is funny now, so why wait? Figure 5–5 relates the five effective emotional strategies to deal with stress.

Figure 5–5
The five effective emotional strategies for combating stress.

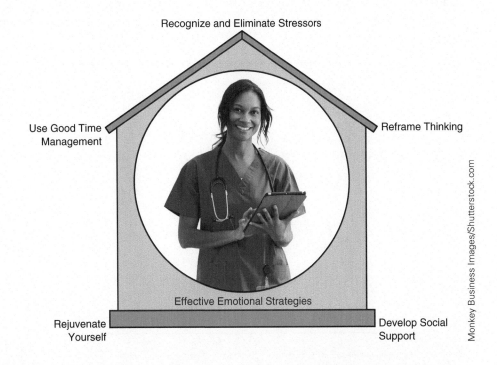

Recognize and Eliminate Stressors

Use Good Time Management

Reframe Thinking

Effective Emotional Strategies

Rejuvenate Yourself

Develop Social Support

Monkey Business Images/Shutterstock.com

Skill Application 5–5 Reframing Your Thinking

The third and final point is to develop effective emotional and physical coping strategies to use when stress gets out of hand. Some may work better for you than others. However, you must develop some on both the physical and emotional sides for balance. This section deals with emotional coping mechanisms.

How you perceive a situation makes all the difference in the world. For each of the following negative perceptions, rewrite in a positive frame of mind.

Example

Negative: *I failed this test, I will never do well in this class!*

Positive: *I failed this test, but I can do better next time and pull my grade up. I will learn from my mistakes and improve my study skills and get a good grade on the next test.*

Negative: *I cannot get along well with others. I will never have any really good friends.*

Positive: _____

Negative: *I do not have any free time to myself. I will never get everything done and have time for me.*

Positive: _____

Negative: *I do not like the way I look.*

Positive: _____

Skill Application 5–6 **Developing a Social Support Group**

Draw a positive picture of yourself, or paste a good photo in the space provided. Now draw several ovals around the picture and write in the names of your social support group. Include teachers, family members, and friends. Your support group may also include members of your community.

Skill Application 5–7 **How Do You Recharge Yourself?**

1. List five things you like to do that take your mind off of stress and make you feel good. Substance abuse does *not* count because we all know that over time, it destroys us and those around us. Remember, the things you choose can do no harm to yourself or others.

   _____

   _____

   _____

   _____

   _____

2. How many times did you do each activity listed in number 1 last week? Place this number next to each activity. Could you have done it more? Can you think of all the excuses why you did not? Remember to take care of yourself and enjoy life so you can truly take care of others.

Effective Physical Strategies

You cannot separate mind from body. If you mentally feel bad, it affects your physical well-being. If you do not take care of your physical body, you lack energy and focus, cannot sleep, and do not reach your full emotional potential. Therefore, you must balance emotional and physical strategies. Indeed, you will see that some of these techniques help both your physical and emotional health. Handling stress "physically" can be broken down into the following four areas:

- Quality sleep and leisure time
- Exercise
- Nutrition
- Relaxation techniques

Quality Sleep and Leisure Time. Adequate sleep is a must for us to function at our peak and handle stress. Research has shown that lack of sleep (sleep deprivation) makes people more susceptible to illness. Of course, lack of sleep also makes people more irritable and less able to focus. Experts recommend that most adults get between 7 and 9 hours of sleep a night.

The quality of sleep is also important. Quality of sleep means you spend most of your sleep cycle in the deeper stages of sleep known as **nonrapid eye movement** or NREM sleep. This is the stage where the body and brain slow down to allow for recharging and regeneration. **Rapid eye movement** or REM sleep is a lighter stage of sleep where you dream and should occupy only a small fraction of your sleep time. Therefore, both quantity (7–8 hours) and quality (majority of time in NREM) sleep are vital to recharging your body. You can enhance your quality of sleep by basically slowing down your mind so that you become able to more quickly get to the deeper stages of sleep. Some suggestions include the following:

- Keep a regular schedule to condition your body to a certain sleep time.
- Reduce noise to the lowest level or substitute noise with recorded soothing sounds.
- Avoid naps as they disrupt your sleep cycle; if you do nap, some advocate no more than 15-minute power naps.
- Keep sleeping area comfortable with as little light as possible.
- Slow down as you get closer to your sleep time and avoid stimulating activity or foods such as chocolate or coffee. Take a soothing bath or meditate to slow your mind and body to ready them for a restful restorative sleep.

Taking leisure time for yourself can also help restore your ability to deal with stress. Even if that leisure time is only 15 minutes, it can help greatly. Sometimes, the more you focus on a major problem, the more stress it causes. This is a good time to take a break and get away from the problem by doing something else. In many cases, the solution will then just come to you as if by magic. It is not magic, just your subconscious mind working for you. This phenomenon is discussed in Chapter 4.

Exercise. Physical exercise and sports are a great way to work off tensions of everyday life. It helps you gain both a physical and mental focus if done properly. Any type of aerobic activity exercises your muscles and relieves mental tension. Vigorous walking, jogging, running, bicycling, and lifting weights are all things you can do by yourself. Of course, you can also find a good workout partner or play team sports. Vigorous exercise also releases a group of hormones called endorphins. These are our body's natural painkillers. They also are mood-elevating chemicals that give us a healthy natural high.

Remember to properly warm up and stretch before any vigorous exercise. You should never stretch "cold" muscles (i.e., muscles that have been inactive). You can march in place, step side to side, or take a walk to warm up your muscles. After the warm-up, you should do your stretches. Stretching not only helps prevent injuries but also helps relieve muscular tension and lower blood pressure. Follow certain rules when stretching. First, never rush through the stretches by bouncing or using fast, jerky movements that could strain or tear muscles. Stretch slowly until you feel mild tension and then hold the position for 10 to 30 seconds.

Nutrition. Good nutrition is a must for our growth and development. It also aids us in fighting stress and disease. In addition, it is a good idea to drink plenty of water. Water makes up most of our body. Water aids in digestion, absorption of nutrients, and removal of waste products. Even though water is found in most foods, you should drink 6 to 8 glasses every day for good health.

Cut down on caffeine, which is found in coffee, tea, and many energy drinks/sodas. Caffeine is a potent central nervous system stimulant. Large amounts can make you anxious, nervous, and unable to get a good night's sleep.

Certain foods have been found to have a calming effect on the body. Foods high in complex carbohydrates (whole grains, beans, seeds, nuts, fruits, and vegetables) have been shown to increase levels of serotonin. Serotonin is a chemical in the brain that helps you feel more relaxed.

Avoid any harmful substances such as illegal drugs, alcohol, or tobacco that can lead to an addictive cycle in dealing with your stress. These substances not only hurt you but also those around you. One example is second-hand or passive smoking where those around you inhale the poisonous substances from the burning cigarette. Another example is drug or alcohol abuse, which can destroy families and relationships. You must be a role model of responsible healthy behaviors for your patients. Imagine how you would feel as a patient if a health care professional entered your room smelling of tobacco and/or alcohol. Most hospitals are smoke free and require smoke-free shifts. Some are even testing hair samples for nicotine and other drugs prior to employment. Your hair holds a long-term record of chemical substance used.

Skill Application 5–8 Assess Your Exercise and Nutrition

Answer the following questions and come up with a plan to improve any no responses.

Example

Do you exercise three times a week for at least 30 minutes each session? *No.*

Plan: *I will develop a schedule that will have three sessions of exercise per week. Because I like to ride my bike, one session will be bicycling for 30 to 40 minutes. This will also help clear my mind.*

1. Do you drink 6 to 8 glasses of drinking water per day?

   Plan: _____

2. Do you follow a good nutritional program?

   Plan: _____

3. Do you eat in moderation?

   Plan: _____

4. Do you limit your caffeine intake?

   Plan: _____

5. Do you avoid substance abuse such as nicotine, alcohol, or illegal street drugs?

   Plan: _____

Relaxation Techniques. Practicing relaxation techniques will help clear your mind and make you sharper. Most people will find a million excuses for why they cannot take the time to relax. Do you see the illogical thinking? If they are that busy, then they need to take the time to relax and restore their body and mind. This time also allows you to listen to your body. Two types of relaxation techniques that are effective are breathing relaxation and meditation techniques.

Slow and deep breathing serves several purposes. First, it increases oxygen to your brain and body. It also slows down your thinking to help clear your head and relax your muscles.

Specific techniques are given at the end of this chapter.

Meditation. **Meditation** techniques can vary greatly. Meditation is basically focusing your attention while clearing your mind of all its constant chattering. You can also use visual or guided imagery to replace troubling thoughts and constant mind chatter with relaxing thoughts and pleasant images. One other related technique is progressive muscle relaxation.

You will get a chance to practice these techniques in the skill application activity at the end of this chapter. Give each a try. You may find some work better for you than others. Practice and use whatever works best for you. These techniques take only 10 to 15 minutes per day, yet they can make your day much more productive. Table 5–2 contrasts some of the dos and don'ts of stress management.

Food for Thought 5–3

Breathing and Stress Reduction

Breathing is something we do automatically, with little or no thought. An individual takes about 20,000 breaths every 24 hours. We are learning that the more we pay attention to our breathing, the better it can help reduce stress. The medical profession and many athletic programs are incorporating ancient yoga breathing techniques in their treatment or training programs.

Yoga breathing is fast becoming a part of mainstream medical practices and is used in stress reduction workshops. Pranayama (pra-nah-YAH-mah), a system of ancient breathing techniques that slows the heart, lowers blood pressure, and relieves stress, has been proven effective.

Yoga breathing teaches you to relax the diaphragm, the main muscle of breathing. Some cardiac rehabilitation programs teach this technique to reduce the stress on the heart and increase oxygen intake from the lungs. In addition, patients with chronic obstructive pulmonary disease (COPD) have been taught this technique to treat their shortness of breath and anxiety when the disease flares up.

Table 5–2
Dos and Don'ts of Stress Management

Do	Don't
Confront a problem	Think it will resolve itself
Discuss things calmly	Fight or yell
Exercise	Lie around, bite nails
Accept responsibility	Blame others
Use relaxation techniques	Use alcohol or drugs
Accept/learn from your mistakes	Be a perfectionist
Keep good nutrition	Overeat or undereat
Be concerned	Worry
Live in the present	Agonize over the past or future
Help others	Avoid people

Skill Application 5–9 Relaxation Techniques

These final activities deal with physical coping mechanisms of stress. This section focuses on some relaxation techniques that will help both your physical and emotional well-being. Try them all and see which ones work best for you. Then devote at least 15 minutes a day using one or more technique. The ideal system is two 15-minute sessions, one in the morning and one before bed.

Practice the following techniques daily for 1 week. Then describe how they make you feel afterward. Keep doing the ones that work best for you.

Technique 1: Breathing Relaxation

1. Lie on a comfortable floor on your back with palms up. Make sure there are no distractions.

2. Now inhale slowly through your nostrils as deeply as you can for 3 to 4 seconds. Fill your lungs, drawing the air in as your abdomen rises. Focus on your abdomen rising and your breathing, and think of nothing else.

3. Hold your breath for 3 to 4 seconds.

4. Then, with your lips slightly open, exhale through your mouth slowly. Breathe normally a few times, and then take another deep breath. Take 10 deep breaths in all.

Describe how you feel: _____

Technique 2: Visual Imagery

Visual imagery is a technique that allows you to picture yourself "relaxed." Visualization or guided imagery is a form of daydreaming.

1. Get in a comfortable position. This can be lying down or in a recliner chair.

2. Close your eyes and take a few deep breaths to calm yourself.

3. Form a clear image in your mind of a pleasant scene, such as a mountaintop, waterfall, or any other place you find relaxing. The idea is to try to engage as many of your senses as possible, imagining the smells, sounds, tastes, and feelings in the scene.

Describe how you feel: _____

Note: A variation of this is to use technique 1, and as you exhale, visually imagine all the stress flowing from your body.

Technique 3: Meditation

Meditation simply means focusing your attention.

1. Again, sit or lie in a comfortable position.

2. Take a slow deep breath (with stomach) and repeat, either aloud or silently, a syllable, a word, or a small group of words that have a positive meaning.

Note: A variation is to gaze at a fixed object, such as a candle, and focus all your thoughts on this object. The key is to not think about anything or to let your mind start talking to you. You can meditate in as little as 5 minutes, although 15 to 20 minutes are optimal for relaxation.

Describe how you feel: _____

(continues)

(continued)

Technique 4: Progressive Relaxation

Progressive muscle relaxation is where you alternately tighten and then relax your muscles. It is a great way to release tension and may even help treat tension headaches.

1. Alternately tense (hold to count of five) and then relax the major muscle groups in your body.

2. Start with your feet, then legs, thighs, buttocks, abdomen, and so on, up to your head.

3. When you release the tension in each group, silently say to yourself, "relax and let go," or use visual imagery to imagine the tension flowing from those muscles.

Describe how you feel: _____

Summary

- Stress is a factor in all our lives. The health care profession can be especially stressful. However, *good stress* can help us perform better, whereas *bad stress* can have a negative impact on our performance.

- Continual high levels of bad stress can lead to several health problems. This chapter discusses a simplified stress management system to use stress as a motivator and an enhancer.

- The first step is to assess and recognize your personal stress signals and stress producers. These can include physical and emotional changes you experience when you have bad stress. By recognizing these signals early, you can quickly develop coping strategies to prevent further stress.

- The second step is to develop specific coping strategies that will work for you. These can include eliminating the stressors you can, reframing your thinking, using good time management techniques, developing a social support group, and taking the time when needed to rejuvenate yourself.

- A third important step is to differentiate the state of worry from being concerned about a situation. To turn worry, which is wasted negative energy, into concern, you must calmly act on the concern.

- Effective physical strategies to help manage your stress include quality sleep and leisure time, exercise, good nutrition, and relaxation techniques.

- Your ability to handle yourself professionally in high stress situations will showcase you as a sought after and trusted professional.

Case Study 5–1

Raheem has an average of two severe tension headaches per week. Having read about stress management, he began to become more aware of his reaction to stress in his life. He noticed that when he began to get "worked up," he would chew on his pencil and a little later his neck muscles would tighten. After a while, his stomach would then get upset, and eventually he would end up with a headache. Do you have any suggestions for Raheem? Do you think he could reduce the number of headaches he experiences? Explain a positive action plan for Raheem that emphasizes early intervention.

_____

_____

_____

_____

_____

Internet Activity

Using Internet search engines, find additional material on stress management that can help you and your fellow students. Some suggested keywords are stress management, harmful effects of stress, depression, worry, meditation, and nutrition. Write down something new that you found to share.

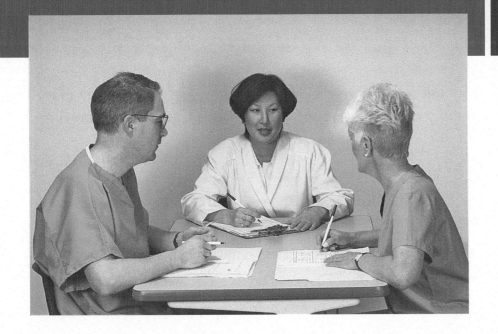

Communicating with Others: Achieving Professional Excellence

This section discusses communication at an interpersonal level within a group, team, or organization. Basic communication skills are stressed, as is their application to success on the job. In addition, this section focuses on job-seeking skills. It emphasizes that the time to prepare for entering the workforce is *right now!* This is why self-assessment and developing specific action plans to showcase your employability potential will be a common theme throughout this book.

You will analyze and build on your strengths. You will also identify areas that need improvement. Chapters covered in this section include the following:

Chapter 6
Types of Communication

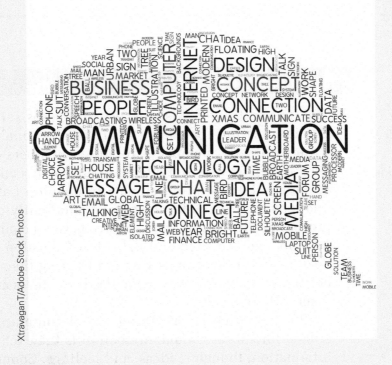

XtravaganT/Adobe Stock Photos

Objectives

Upon completion of this chapter, you should be able to:

1. Describe the essential ingredients of the communication process.

2. Contrast the various types of nonverbal communication.

3. Explain the various types of verbal communication.

4. Describe the components of effective written communication.

5. Describe methods to maximize verbal, nonverbal, and written communication.

Key Terms

clear message	encoding	oral communication
colloquial language	enunciation	pronunciation
communication	feedback	receiver
communication process	jargon	sender
decodes	lay language	verbal communication
electronic communication	nonverbal communication	written communication

Introduction

A word is dead when it is said, some say. I say it just begins to live that day.

—Emily Dickinson

The first section of this worktext discusses self-communication. Communication for a health care professional must occur with patients, family members, and other members of the health care team to deliver safe and effective care. Good communication skills allow health care professionals to develop better interpersonal relations with patients, coworkers, and family members and help prevent medical errors from occurring. Good communication makes patients feel accepted and helps them develop confidence in the health care professionals who are treating them. Communication helps professionals identify the needs of others and determine how to meet those needs.

But just what is this thing called communication that is so crucial for success? **Communication** is the exchange of messages, information, thoughts, ideas, and feelings. Communication can be in **verbal**, **nonverbal**, or **written/electronic** form. Verbal communication is primarily the spoken word, such as in conversations, oral reports, voice mail, telephone messages, and speeches. Nonverbal communication includes behavior such as facial expressions, gestures, body language, symbols, and touch. Written and electronic communication include such items as memos, letters, reports, charts/electronic medical records, e-mail, text messages, and video and computer transfer of information.

Anticipatory Exercise 6–1 One- and Two-Way Communication

This chapter will discuss the importance of feedback in the communication process. However, sometimes feedback does not occur because of the pattern of the communication process. For example, in one-way communication, the sender transmits a message, and once the receiver gets it, the process is complete and feedback does not occur. When you receive junk mail or spam e-mail and simply throw it away or delete it, one-way communication has taken place.

(continues)

(continued)

List three other examples of one-way communication, either personal or professional.

a. _____

b. _____

c. _____

Two-way communication occurs when the sender transmits a message, the receiver gets it, and there is some type of feedback or response. Conversations are examples of two-way communication, provided that more than one individual does the talking. Of course, if one individual monopolizes the conversation, they are probably going to receive nonverbal cues such as rolling of the eyes or tapping of an object or foot as feedback.

List five different examples of two-way communication.

a. _____

b. _____

c. _____

d. _____

e. _____

Types of Messages

Information or messages can be conveyed by various means. List three examples for each message type, along with an advantage and disadvantage for each.

Example

Written message: *letter; advantage: can be personal in nature; disadvantage: takes time to send and receive*

Types of Messages

1. a. Written 1: _____

   b. Written 2: _____

   c. Written 3: _____

2. a. Verbal 1: _____

   b. Verbal 2: _____

   c. Verbal 3: _____

3. a. Nonverbal 1: _____

   b. Nonverbal 2: _____

   c. Nonverbal 3: _____

Overview of the Communication Process

An effective **communication process** has four basic ingredients: a **sender**, a **clear message**, a **receiver**, and a mechanism for **feedback**.

Although the process of communication seems simple, it is one of the most difficult tasks that humans perform. The process begins with the sender. The sender is the person who transmits the message. The sender begins the process by creating a message that they want to convey. The receiver is the person for whom the message is intended. A mechanism for feedback can ensure effective communication because it can confirm that the sender and the receiver have the same understanding of the message that was sent. Figure 6–1 shows the basic elements needed for effective communication.

Let us now take a more in-depth look at this delicate process. The sender is the originator of the idea or message that is to be conveyed. The sender must choose the best way to convert the idea(s) or message(s) into words, diagrams, graphs, reports, and so on. This conversion process is called **encoding** the message. It may be that the sender decides that a memo is the best way to encode a particular thought. In turn, another thought may be best encoded in a personal letter format or sent via e-mail. Each situation must be assessed to determine the most effective way to encode and transfer the thoughts of the sender.

The message that is sent needs to be clearly understood by everyone who receives it. The receiver **decodes** the message, which means that they interpret the message. Because messages reach our ears and eyes (body language), it is important that interruptions and distractions be kept at a minimum.

Another important factor in effective communication is making sure that the message is in terms that both the sender and receiver understand. This is especially true for health care professionals because we have our own language, called medical terminology. This terminology is often not understood by others not in the health care field.

Figure 6–1
Basic elements necessary for effective communication.

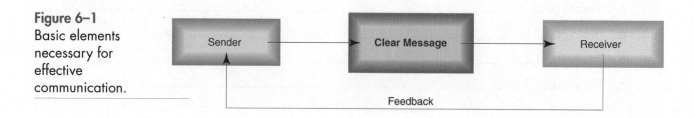

Food **for** Thought 6–1

Special Considerations When Communicating with Patients

Now that you understand the basics of the communication process, what special considerations need to be taken into account in the health care setting? For example, what about patients who are sensory deprived (hearing or vision loss) or heavily medicated? What about patients who can hear but cannot respond because of medications, medical equipment, or disease process? Some patients cannot speak because they have a tube inserted through their voice box (larynx) leading into their lungs. What special considerations are appropriate for these individuals? Can you

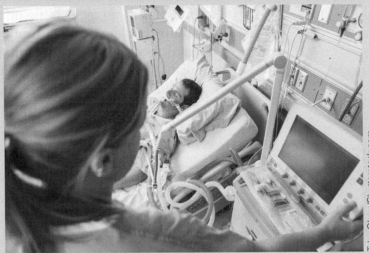

Figure 6–2
Can you identify difficulties in communicating with this patient?

think of any more special circumstances in health care that can impair communication? Refer to Figure 6–2 and identify possible difficulties in communicating with the patient.

You should also avoid slang words or words with double meanings; we sometimes refer to these words as **jargon**. For example, the word *expire* means to breathe out or exhale. Expire can also mean to die. Therefore, when instructing a patient, it may not be a good idea to say, "I want you to expire now." It would be better to simply say breathe out or exhale. Meaningless terms such as *like, you know, all that stuff, um,* and *okay* distract from the main message you are trying to convey and should be avoided.

Feedback is an often-neglected part of the communication process. The receiver should provide the sender with feedback to show how well the message was received and understood. This can be done in several ways. For example, the receiver can ask questions for clarification, give answers, or react by doing something that demonstrates how well (or poorly) the message was understood. The sender now knows that the message was indeed received and now has some insights about the receiver's interpretation, or decoding.

Once feedback is received, the sender may choose to clarify the message by repeating it or changing the form. In addition, the sender may request further feedback and clarification from the receiver.

Often, patients are the receivers of our messages. Patients may hear messages, but they may not fully understand them because of the unfamiliar terms or just simply because of the environment, which is unfamiliar and sometimes intimidating. Patients receiving bad news may feel overwhelmed with emotion, which in turn limits their ability to receive the information. Many people do not want to admit that they do not understand terms being used because they think health care professionals will perceive them as "dumb." The health care professional should ask questions that require the patient to demonstrate understanding. Simple yes or no questions are not appropriate. The health care professional may need to rephrase the explanation until they are sure that the patient understands.

Just For

FUN 6–1

Explaining Medical Jargon

Listed below are some medical terms. Attempt to explain them to a classmate in lay (everyday) terminology. *Hint:* A medical terminology book or medical dictionary will be of great assistance to you.

Atelectasis   Bradycardia

Osteoporosis   Laparoscopy

Hysterectomy   Rhinoplasty

Rhinitis   Cholecystectomy

Skill Application 6–1 Feedback

Pick a simple procedure to explain to another student. This could be a procedure such as how to properly take a pulse or blood pressure, or it could be some form of patient education concerning a disease process. Record your explanation and interaction, and then play it back and evaluate its effectiveness. For example, did you clarify points when they were not understood? Did you use slang or meaningless terminology? Give a written critique of your performances, listing the positive and negative aspects.

1. Positive: _____

_____

_____

_____

2. Negative: _____

_____

_____

_____

_____

(continues)

(continued)

Communication Distortion (The Gossip Game)

Gather a group of at least eight students together in a circle. Have one person start by whispering the following story to the person next to them. Continue doing this until the last person in the group has heard the story. Have this person state the story out loud to the group and then have the first person read the original story. Now compare the results. What did you find? List some of your conclusions.

Story

A patient was brought into the ER with multiple chest trauma from a vehicular accident. The patient was experiencing SOB and had tachycardia with low blood pressure. The patient was rushed to the OR, where a right pneumothorax was found and repaired. He spent two days in the ICU and then went to a general care floor. He eventually made a complete recovery and was discharged from the hospital.

Conclusions:_____

_____

_____

_____

Types of Communication

Nonverbal Communication

Nature gave you your face, but you must provide the expression.

— Author Unknown

There are three basic types of communication. Nonverbal communication consists mainly of body language, whereas verbal communication is usually the spoken word; the last form is written communication. Our discussion begins with a focus on nonverbal communication.

Nonverbal communication makes up most of the human communication and may be even more effective than verbal communication. Surprisingly, studies of face-to-face communication show that 80% to 90% of the impact of a message comes from nonverbal elements. These elements include facial expressions, eye contact, body language, touch, personal space, and appearance.

Facial Expressions. Many say that a smile is the universal language. The face is a portal that can reflect many of our thoughts and feelings as we are presenting a message. Besides smiles, we can have frowns, scowls, glares, puzzled looks, and so on.

Eye Contact. Smiles convey a message of friendliness around the world, but eye contact does not. In some cultures, looking downward while speaking is a sign of respect, whereas in the United States, this action may be interpreted as meaning that the messenger has something to hide. However, eye contact is important when talking to patients because it lets them know that you are paying attention.

Body Language. Do you know someone who talks with their hands? Do you talk with your hands? We all use body language, whether it is in the form of hands flailing, feet shuffling, finger tapping, head nodding, shoulder shrugging, and so on. Body language can send some powerful signals about how we feel. Body posture is also part of body language. The way you carry yourself while standing or sitting transmits nonverbal messages. For example, someone who maintains their body in an upright position with shoulders up and head held high conveys confidence. An individual who walks around slouched over with shoulders and head down conveys a message of sadness and unhappiness.

When interacting with a patient, it is important to lean forward during a conversation to convey the message, "I am interested." If you stand too stiff or tall, you may appear tense or uninterested. Crossing your arms can show an unwillingness to accept what the patient has to say.

Touch. Health care professionals use touch to convey compassion and concern. Unfortunately, touch can also take the form of physical and sexual abuse. It is important for health care professionals to contrast proper and improper touch. A brief hug, a hand squeeze, or a pat on the back can convey a message of compassion. You should always ask your patient permission to touch; you can simply say, "Would it be okay if I held your hand, you seem upset?"

If the touch has any suggestion of sexual or physical abuse, it is highly improper. Examples of improper and unacceptable forms of touch include patting, slapping, pinching, and stroking of a patient's buttocks or various body parts. In fact, any unwanted touch could be perceived as abuse.

Personal Space or Distance. We also communicate by how little or how much distance we allow between the sender and the receiver. People who know each other well are usually comfortable within a foot of each other. However, to have a stranger in your face, so to speak, would most likely make you uncomfortable because they have invaded your personal space. People who do not know each other well usually stand 4 to 12 feet apart when they first communicate with each other.

Physical presence, such as bending over someone while trying to communicate, can be intimidating. A patient may perceive this as a stature associated with power and authority and can become intimidated. This is why it is sometimes helpful to sit by the bedside at the patient's level. In the office setting, you can sit in a chair alongside the patient, avoid only looking at your computer and not the patient.

Appearance. The way we dress and groom ourselves also sends out powerful messages. Would you have much confidence in a health care professional who entered your room in cutoff jeans and a tank top and whose hair obviously had not been washed in days? It makes no difference how competent this individual may be. The nonverbal message that the person cannot care for themself has been sent, and most would interpret this to mean that the person also cannot care for patients. Your appearance has a great effect on your ability to get your message across. Places of employment have dress codes and standards. Make sure you adhere to those standards. Refer to Figure 6–3 and choose the better nonverbal image.

Figure 6–3
Which nonverbal message is better?

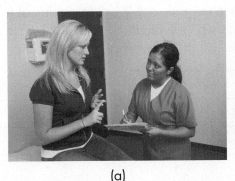 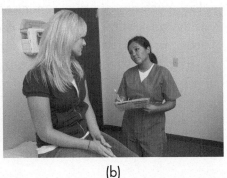

(a)   (b)

Test Yourself 6–1

Nonverbal Communication

What would the following nonverbal communications mean to you if you were the patient interacting with a health care professional who gave these nonverbal messages? Give a brief statement of how you would feel after each gesture.

1. Purposeful silence: _____
2. Handshake: _____
3. Shrug of the shoulder: _____
4. Indirect eye contact: _____
5. Frown: _____
6. Yawn: _____
7. Finger tapping: _____
8. Raised eyebrows: _____
9. One raised eyebrow: _____
10. Pursed lips: _____
11. Facial tension: _____

Food for Thought 6–2

First Impressions

It may sound corny, but you never get a second chance to make a good first impression. Think about that. If your patients' first impression of you is poor, do you think they will comply with the treatment or have faith in your abilities? Can you think of some examples of nonverbal communication that would enhance a favorable first impression and, therefore, be the first step in establishing a trusting patient–caregiver relationship? As a start, what about good posture and hygiene? Can you think of more?

Skill Application 6–2 Observing Nonverbal Communication

How much nonverbal communication do you use? Work in groups of three. Designate one person as the observer/recorder. The other two individuals will have a 10-minute conversation, while the observer records (out of their sight) all the nonverbal communication used in the conversation. Switch roles so that everyone gets the chance to be an observer.

Observations: _____

_____

_____

_____

Mixed Messages
(When Verbal and Nonverbal Messages Disagree)

Nonverbal communication is said to be more powerful than the spoken words. Have you ever heard someone say, "It wasn't what he said, but how he said it"? Nonverbal communication is difficult to control, and any communication that is not consistent sends a mixed message to the patient. A mixed message occurs when the verbal message is saying one thing and the nonverbal message is saying another, causing a direct conflict.

For example, suppose that a health care professional says, "I'm really excited about the progress in your recovery, you're doing great." However, while saying this, the person had a sad and tense-looking face and the shoulders were slumped forward. Do you think the message was genuine? Would this inspire confidence and trust in that patient?

Have students work in pairs developing a short skit that shows a mixed message. One example could be a therapist and patient in a room where the patient is very concerned about their treatment and is asking questions. The therapist says that they are concerned but frequently checks the time, rolls their eyes, taps a foot, or stares out the window.

Describe your skit and the mixed messages.

_____

_____

_____

Verbal Communication

Instructions and information can be presented to patients, coworkers, and visitors verbally, nonverbally, and even with various audiovisual methods. We have already discussed nonverbal communication, so now we will explore verbal communication in more detail. Verbal communication uses words to convey the message.

In the health care setting, you will use words to explain procedures to your patients and to record and report your observations. Make sure that the terms and concepts that you are presenting are in a language that the listener can understand. You must choose your words carefully so that your message is clear and understandable.

Oral Communication. Oral communication is the form of communication we use most often. This is our conversation with our peers, friends, patients, fellow health care professionals, or family members. This form of communication does not always have to be face-to-face. An example would be when you use a cell phone or other forms of communication during which you can hear but not see the person on the other end.

Face-to-face discussions provide the best opportunity for the exchange of information, points of view, and instructions, while providing immediate feedback. This feedback can be in the form of return oral communication (questions) or nonverbal cues such as a puzzled look. This can immediately relay signals to the sender that further explanation and clarification are needed.

Several factors enter into the effectiveness of oral communication. These include the manner and tone of your voice, the language used, and nonverbal signals.

Manner and Tone of Voice. The *tone* and *manner* of a message can convey excitement, anger, disappointment, cheerfulness, and so on. Your tone of voice reveals your feelings and attitudes. Because tone of voice is so revealing, you should be aware of what you sound like. Remember, it is not always what you say but how you say it.

The tone, volume, and inflection of your voice can detract from or add to your message. You can either stimulate or calm a patient merely with your voice and behavior. Your voice can have several characteristics, including volume, pitch, and rate.

The volume of your voice refers to its intensity or loudness. In most situations, a moderate volume is appropriate unless the patient has certain characteristics that limit their ability to hear you. In addition, when providing a group of patients with education, it is more than likely that you will have to raise the volume of your voice for everyone to hear. A good speaker will be able to use volume changes or inflection to emphasize certain parts of the message that they believe to be particularly important.

Pitch refers to whether you have a high- or low-pitched voice. People who speak with a high-pitched voice sound shrill and whiny. Conversely, if your voice is too low pitched, you may be hard to understand. Again, moderation is the key. A moderate pitch with variations is best for standard speech.

Rate is the speed at which you speak. A moderate rate is again best, with some variation so as not to be boring. You can vary your rate by slowing down to emphasize main points or pausing to allow the receiver to reflect on what you said.

Language Used. As a health care professional, you want to be perceived as intelligent, caring, and competent. Your speech can add to or detract from this perception. You should always attempt to speak clearly and concisely and avoid meaningless sounds or message distracters such as *like*, *um*, *uh*, and *okay*.

Every day, or **lay, language**, is the best when explaining concepts or procedures to patients and family members. For example, say you need to assess a patient's breath sounds. When explaining the procedure to the patient, you should say something such as, "I'm going to listen to how well your lungs sound" versus "I'm going to auscultate your pulmonary system to assess for any adventitious breath sounds." Although the second statement may impress the patient, it will add distance to establishing trust and communication. Lay language is not to be mistaken for informal or **colloquial language**. Colloquial language is informal words and phrases such as "sleep tight" or "don't cause a ruckus." Informal language is used between friends and family members, never with patients.

Last, it is also important for you to pronounce words accurately, enunciate (speak clearly), and use good vocabulary and correct grammar.

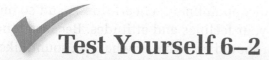

Test Yourself 6–2

Enunciation versus Pronunciation

Enunciation refers to the clarity with which you say words. Saying *didja* for *did you* or *gimme* for *give me* are examples of poor enunciation. Poor enunciation is the result of leaving out sounds, adding sounds, and/or running sounds together, all of which can confuse patients and may diminish your status among coworkers.

Following is a list of some common terms that are poorly enunciated. Can you identify what the term is? Also, do you properly enunciate the term?

Whacha want.

Goin to the pon to go fishin.

I read the lil pome.

Praps what I said was crul.

C'mere, woodja an gimmee your hand.

(continues)

(continued)

Pronunciation is closely related to enunciation. Pronunciation refers to the correctness with which you say words. You are not just running words together or leaving out a letter or two as with enunciation; you are saying the word wrong by mispronouncing it. What is the correct term or pronunciation for the following?

Omost _____   Famly _____

Liberry _____   Burgular _____

Kindeegarden _____   Corps _____

Idear _____   Jest _____

Sophmore _____   Preventive _____

Nonverbal Signals

Observation of patients' nonverbal messages will tell you whether they understand or are even listening to your message. This is another reason why it is important to maintain good eye contact with your receiver. As stated earlier, posture can send powerful nonverbal messages along with the conversation. Sitting behind a large desk or in an imposing chair or standing over the person with whom you are conversing sends a message that you are powerful and dominant. An environment that contributes to a relaxed atmosphere and has minimal or no outside distractions is most conducive for effective communication. Pay attention to the mannerisms and posture of your patients. These will tell you how they are receiving your verbal message. Are they slouched over, head down, tapping their foot, doodling on paper, and so on?

Finally, listening is a crucial part of oral communication. So much so that listening is developed more fully in Chapter 7. For now, remember that nothing conveys your interest more in the other person than listening carefully. A conversation is a two-way communication, and you must listen for feedback to make it fully effective. If you monopolize the conversation and do not let others talk, you are also sending the message that what they have to say is not important. Always remember how good it feels when someone is truly listening to you.

Skill Application 6–3 Tone and Manner of Speech

How you say something can greatly change its intended meaning. Working in pairs, practice saying the following statements exactly as they are provided, but vary your tone to convey excitement, disappointment, anger, and so on. See if the receiver can pick the correct emotion.

Statement   **Emotion**

There is a fire in the room.   _____

You did that procedure well.   _____

I think everything will be all right.   _____

(continues)

(continued)

I like talking to you.

_____

Your lab tests turned out well.

_____

No, I don't mind doing that for you.

_____

Mirroring a Conversation

When you have a conversation, you can mirror the speech and nonverbal actions of your receiver. Mirroring a conversation means that it becomes a reflection of itself. For example, you can match the pace, pitch, tone, volume, posture, or nonverbal messages of the other person. This gives the other person a sense of oneness or connectedness with you and may help them relax and open up to you. Be careful not to mirror everything to the point that it looks like you are mimicking or mocking the individual. The pace of a conversation is usually a good area to control.

For example, if you are talking to someone who speaks very slowly, mirror their pace and gradually speed that person up without making them aware of it. If you sense that someone is tense, slowly relax your posture and keep your voice calm and facial expressions pleasant. See if this causes the person to relax. You cannot work in pairs with mirroring because the other person cannot be aware of what you are doing. Therefore, practice this technique at home or with friends. Start by seeing if you can alter the pace of the conversation. Experiment and record and share your observations.

Observations: _____

_____

_____

_____

_____

Self-Assessment

Working in groups of three, have each member do a self-assessment and rate each of the following questions as never, always, or sometimes. Then, pick an observer and have the other two members engage in a 10-minute conversation. The observer will rate the other two on a separate sheet of paper in each of the categories. Use examples as much as possible to justify your ratings. Recording the conversations could be beneficial. Continue until everyone gets a chance to rate the others and compare results.

Note: Standard English is the English spoken by news broadcasters, which is free of regional accents. For example, they would not use the western Pennsylvania term *youns*, meaning you all, nor would they speak with a southern drawl and say *y'all.*

1. I speak standard English. _____

2. I speak at a moderate volume. _____

3. I speak at a moderate pitch. _____

4. I speak at a moderate rate. _____

(continues)

(continued)

5. I periodically vary my volume, rate, and pitch for emphasis of main points and to maintain interest. _____

6. I use pauses to emphasize major points. _____

7. I enunciate clearly. _____

8. I use proper pronunciations. _____

9. I use appropriate body language and gestures. _____

10. I use correct grammar. _____

Written Communication

In oral communication, no permanent record of what has been said exists. People may forget or even distort part of the message. Although oral communication is used more often, written messages are indispensable and are especially important in health care activities. Written messages are also a more formal means of communication. A well-balanced communication system includes both written and oral communication.

Written communication should be similar to oral communication in that it should be concise and should use understandable language. It is also important that you use proper grammar and ensure that every word is spelled correctly. Diagrams, graphs, drawings, or photographs can be used to show a specific sequence of events or to aid in the understanding of difficult concepts. In addition, films, videos, DVDs, and interactive computer programs can be useful to educate or instruct a patient or family members.

Written messages provide a record that can be accessed and referred to as often as necessary. In addition, written communication can contain better-organized and researched information because you can take the necessary time to organize your thoughts. You can also reread, edit, and redraft your thoughts until you are satisfied with the final document. Written communication is preferred when important details are involved and a permanent record is necessary such as a patient's chart or record. As a health care professional, you will use written communication often. Some examples are as follows:

- Taking or giving messages and orders
- Writing notes on patients' charts
- Writing policies and procedures
- Developing patient educational material
- Writing memos or letters

Food **for** Thought 6–3

When Does It Need to Be "in Writing"?

Sometimes it is important to follow up an oral conversation or even a confrontation with a written message. A written message may need to follow as a reminder of orally agreed-upon duties. For example, if you are a supervisor and request certain tasks of an individual with a certain deadline, you should put this in writing for your sake and the employee's sake.

A written message can also follow an oral communication of a job well done. This way the employee has a positive permanent record to keep on file. Can you think of other instances in which a written message should follow an oral communication?

Writing a Message

The first step in writing any message, regardless of its form, is to determine whether it is necessary. Ask yourself, "Can I deliver this message as well if not better by telephone or a face-to-face conversation? Do I need a permanent record of this message for legal or disciplinary actions?"

The second step is to decide what format your message will take. Will it be a letter, e-mail, or memo? Will it be in report form? A memo or e-mail usually is internal in nature; that is, they stay within the organization. A letter usually is sent outside of an organization. A report can be either internally or externally circulated. Text messaging is a short and casual type of written communication. Abbreviations, slang, and jargon are used. It is imperative that you write memos, letters, and e-mails using appropriate grammar, spelling, and punctuation. Be very careful not to apply your texting language to formal communications.

The final step involves the actual writing process. Always consider the five Ws when writing a message:

Who is the primary reader, and who should get copies?

What are you trying to accomplish? What do you want the reader to do? What is fact, and what is opinion? What do the readers already know? What questions are they likely to have? What do you want to avoid?

Why is this important or interesting to the reader?

When will the things happen, and when are the deadlines?

Where will things happen? Where can additional information be obtained?

Figure 6–4 shows the five Ws of a memo.

Figure 6–4
Five Ws of a memo.

To: (**W**hom) William Smith, Chairperson
From: (**W**hom) Mary Jones, Surgical Technologist
Subject: (**W**hy) Important meeting
Date: (**W**hen) October 1, 2024

          (**W**hat) This memo is to inform you of an
                      upcoming organization meeting for
                      the Allied Health Committee.
          (**W**here) The meeting will take place at the
                      board room of the Administration
                      Building
          (**W**hen) at 10:00 a.m. Nov. 15, 2024.
                      Please RSVP if you can attend.
                      Look forward to seeing you there.

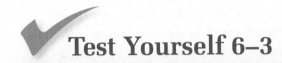

Test Yourself 6–3

Preparing a First Rough Draft

Your health care club is preparing to do a charity walk to benefit cystic fibrosis. You are in charge of soliciting donations from local businesses. Write a sample letter that will be attached to an e-mail requesting donations.

Prepare a rough draft using a free flow of thought. This means to simply write as if you are talking. Use your notes on the five Ws and any other critical information that needs to be included. Do not worry about spelling, grammar, and punctuation at this time. Do not worry about your terminology; write the first thought that comes to mind.

Now, review your rough draft, and begin to organize it, trying to keep the reader's perspective in mind. Select an opening statement carefully. This statement is what the reader remembers best, so make sure that it clearly states your main point. Make it an attention grabber by using startling statistics, questions, or something that especially interests the reader.

Rewrite the rest of the message making it short, personal, and to the point. Check each paragraph to make sure that it has a major thought. Each paragraph should flow into the next paragraph and can be linked by words such as *furthermore*, *consequently*, and *in addition to*.

Prepare your closing statement. This is what the readers remember second best, so it should include some statement about where or whom to contact for further questions or comments, and so on.

Finally, double-check your grammar, spelling, and terminology. You should have no errors in your document. Remember, word processing has good spell-checking programs and a thesaurus to improve the vocabulary. However, when using the thesaurus, remember that although the suggested words may have similar meanings to your original word, they may not have identical meanings. Therefore, it is important that you choose only those words that you fully understand, or you might end up saying something other than what you intended. Also remember that spell checks will not pick up unintended words that are correctly spelled. For example, if you type "form" and meant to type "from," the spell checker will recognize form as correctly spelled and not alert you. Always have at least one person read your draft before you send it out.

The last step will be to draft the text of the e-mail to which this letter will be attached. Devise a subject line that will spark enough interest from the recipient to open the attachment.

Summary

- By learning about the communication process, you can take the first step in becoming an effective communicator.
- Communication is one of the most powerful skills you will ever possess and use.
- Communication is the exchange of messages, information, thoughts, ideas, and feelings. It requires a sender, a clear message, a receiver, and some mechanism for feedback.
- Health care professionals need to take special care in assessing patient's understanding of the message being sent. There are many barriers to receiving a clear message when you are ill.
- Communication can be nonverbal, verbal, or written.
- Nonverbal communication includes facial expressions, eye contact, body language, touch, personal space, and appearance.
- Verbal communication includes manner, tone of voice, and the use and selection of language.
- Written communication includes letters, memos, and e-mails and provides a permanent record of the conversation.
- The communication process is complex and multifactorial. There can be a breakdown in many different areas. It is important to recognize communication errors and attempt to correct them immediately. In future chapters, we will discuss barriers to communication in more depth.

Case Study 6–1

Joliene was about to begin her first clinical experience. She was an above-average student and always did well on her written exams. She studied hard but kept to herself and was very shy. The teacher noticed that she did not make eye contact or smile in class or lab. Joliene always did extra credit and volunteered whenever there were written assignments. Her papers were always outstanding.

What are Joliene's communication strengths?

_____

_____

_____

_____

_____

What are Joliene's communication weaknesses?

_____

_____

_____

_____

_____

(continues)

(continued)

Give an action plan that Joliene should utilize prior to attending her clinical rotations to make it a positive experience.

_____

_____

_____

_____

_____

Internet Activity

Using Internet search engines, find additional information on the position of the Institutes of Medicine (IOM) on the connection between communication and medical errors. Suggested search words include Institutes of Medicine, to err is human, and medical errors. Write down something new that you found to share.

_____

_____

_____

_____

_____

Chapter 7
Communication in Action

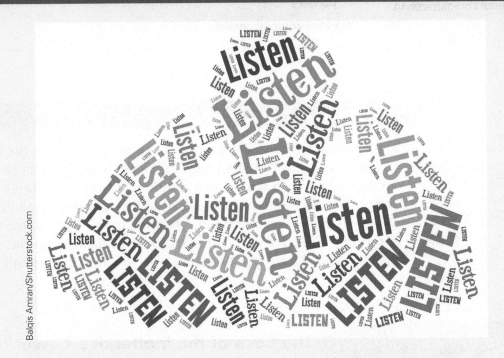

Balqis Amran/Shutterstock.com

Objectives

Upon completion of this chapter, you should be able to:

1. Assess environmental and personal barriers to the communication process.

2. Describe effective methods to break down your defined barriers.

3. Develop optimal listening skills and use these skills to maximize your communication potential.

4. Develop good customer relations skills.

5. Develop effective public speaking skills.

Key Terms

active listening

close-ended questions

complacency

customer relations

environmental communication
    barriers

hearing

listening

open-ended questions

personal communication
    barriers

selective comprehension

selective memory

semantic barriers

telephone etiquette

Introduction

I learn a great deal by merely observing you, and letting you talk as long as you please, and taking note of what you do not say.

—T. S. Eliot

Understanding the various types of communications is the first step in becoming an effective communicator. Now we need to look at communication in action in a dynamic system. Are there barriers within us and the environment that inhibit effective communication? Why is listening so important, yet often overlooked in the communication process? Why is effective communication important to an organization? These questions and more are answered in this chapter.

Anticipatory Exercise 7–1   The Case of the Inattentive Coworker

You are a night-shift supervisor at a small community hospital. Each night, during report, you distribute and explain staff workloads. One of the employees is always interrupting, chatting about other topics, or just not paying attention. The employee has made a lot of little mistakes in the past and constantly needs to be retold what to do.

1. Why does this employee function poorly?

_____

2. What can you do as a supervisor to improve this employee's work performance?

_____

Barriers to Communication

Barriers to communication can be either environmental or personal in nature. The environmental barriers include everything outside of the individual that can inhibit communication. For example, excessive noise or poor comfort conditions would impair effective communication. The personal barriers include what is within the individuals who are communicating. These may include emotions, attitude, and prejudices.

Environmental Barriers

The environment can either enhance or detract from the communication process. **Environmental communication barriers** can also be called physical factors.

Noise. If a room is noisy, it will impair the speaker and listener's ability to communicate. Have you ever heard someone say, "It's so noisy, I can't hear myself think"? Noise levels should be kept at a minimal level. For example, a noisy treatment room can cause not only distraction but also increased patient anxiety levels.

Activity Levels. If there is a lot of other activity around you, it is easy to become distracted and unable to fully focus on the communication process. Excessive amounts of visual stimulation lessen our ability to fully use our sense of hearing. Have you heard that some blind or visually impaired people may develop a keener sense of hearing?

Physical Arrangement. How the furniture is arranged can make a difference. Think how you would feel sitting around a small circular table in comfortable chairs communicating with patients. Now picture yourself in front of a large imposing podium on a stage talking down to patients seated in neat rows at hard desks. Which physical arrangement is more conducive for patient education? Physical arrangement should also allow for a private place to talk when needed.

Comfort Levels. If you are physically uncomfortable, it will be difficult for your mental processes to work at peak function. Can you concentrate in a room that is too hot or cold? What if you are uncomfortable sitting or standing while communicating with a patient? Do you think that person may pick up on nonverbal signals showing your discomfort? What if the patient interprets this as a lack of concern? Comfort levels are important for both the receiver and the sender.

Technological Barriers. These can include inadequate telephone capabilities. For example, what if you have a poor connection? This would certainly interfere with optimal communication. Another example is a DVD or recorded lecture for patient education. What if they will not play, the sound is not working, or the image is poor? Again, this will cause communication to be impaired because of a technological barrier. Computer viruses, errors in e-mail transmissions, or interruptions in Internet service are becoming more common technological barriers as we increasingly rely on electronic communication.

Figure 7-1
Environmental barriers to communication.

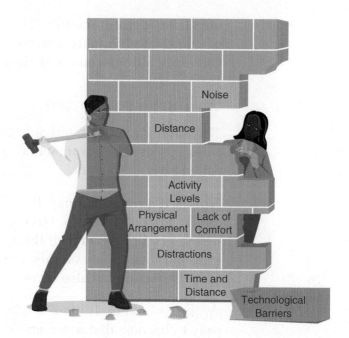

Time and Distance. An excessive distance between people can act as a barrier. Imagine standing far away from a patient with hearing difficulties. Getting too close and making a patient or coworker uncomfortable by invading their personal space can also inhibit communication. The time available to communicate must be adequate to allow for an effective transmission of the message and feedback to occur. Figure 7-1 shows environmental barriers to communication.

Personal Barriers

Personal communicational barriers exist within yourself or the person with whom you are communicating. Personal barriers are sometimes not quite as obvious as environmental barriers. Personal barriers can include the following.

Emotional Barriers. Feelings and emotions create barriers to communication. Stress, fear, anger, and sadness can all make it difficult to concentrate on the communication. Even positive emotions, such as love and happiness, can also prevent effective communication. For example, someone who just won the lottery or found the love of a lifetime may have trouble focusing on ordinary conversations.

Attitudes. Certain attitudes can impair communication. For example, prejudices toward people, because of their religion, race, or membership in a group, is a communication barrier. Racial and ethnic groups are often the targets of prejudice. People can also have negative attitudes toward older adults, women, men, people with low incomes, people with disabilities, and people with different lifestyles. You must identify and overcome any type of prejudice that you may have to effectively communicate with coworkers and patients who are representative of various groups.

Another type of attitude that acts as a barrier is **selective comprehension**. This is when people focus on the part of the conversation that interests them the most and pay little attention to everything else. Have you ever heard someone say, "You're only hearing what you want to hear"?

Related to this is **selective memory**, when we tend to remember certain things (usually the positive) and forget other things. For example, we may remember and focus on all the procedures we performed well, but we may be "fuzzy" concerning the ones at which we were weak.

Complacency, or indifference, is another attitude that blocks communication. This is the "I don't care attitude." Here, even if the message may get through, it may be acted on only half-heartedly or not at all.

Language. Words can create a barrier to communication. What if your patient speaks another language? Even if you are both speaking the same language, people do not understand each other for many reasons. For example, often a health care professional will use highly technical language when explaining a technique to a patient. Instead, it is best to use plain, simple words and direct, uncomplicated language that the patient can relate to and understand what you are saying. This is called *lay language* (see Figure 7–2).

Resistance to Change. Have you ever heard someone say, "This is the way we've always done things around here"? Resistance to change is quite common and can be a serious barrier to communication. Resistance to change can occur because many communications may be conveying the message that a new idea, assignment, or change in the daily familiar routine is now warranted without any explanation why. Many people are comfortable with the familiar and prefer things to stay the way they are, which is why it is critical to convey the reason for the change. This will allow people to accept it better.

Figure 7–2
Use lay person terminology to be sure your patients understand what you are saying.

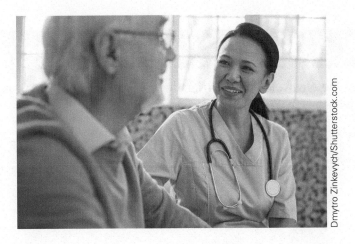

Dmytro Zinkevych/Shutterstock.com

Just For FUN 7-1

Many Meanings

Many words in our language can have similar meanings depending on how they are used, the tone of voice, and so on. Match the word from List A to a word with a similar meaning in List B. Which list has a negative connotation?

List A
1. _____ Firm
2. _____ Aggressive
3. _____ Compassionate
4. _____ Easygoing
5. _____ Confident
6. _____ Detail Person
7. _____ Direct

List B
a. Cocky
b. Ruthless
c. Tactless
d. Unconcerned
e. Unyielding
f. Picky
g. Bleeding Heart

Answers can be found in Appendix F.

Food for Thought 7-1

Special Patient Circumstances

Patients will often present you with special circumstances. For each of the circumstances described, tell what kind of special communication skills you would use.

1. Patient is confused.
2. Patient speaks a different language.
3. Patient is blind.
4. Patient is hearing impaired.
5. Patient can understand but cannot speak. This is termed aphasia (a = without, phasia = speech).
6. Patient has just learned that they have a terminal illness.

Skill Application 7-1 Assessing Environmental Barriers

Assess the environmental barriers in your classroom, home, or place of employment. List three barriers with suggested improvements.

Barrier 1: _____

Suggested improvement: _____

_____

Barrier 2: _____

(continues)

(continued)

Suggested improvement: _____

_____

Barrier 3: _____

Suggested improvement: _____

_____

Assessing Personal Barriers

The effective caregiver is aware of and able to identify personal attitudes or prejudices that may interfere with their ability to effectively communicate. Once identified, the prejudices can be reduced or even eliminated. This awareness, honest assessment, and the subsequent action to overcome these conditions will make you an excellent communicator.

List two attitudes or prejudices that you have to work on improving. Remember, attitudes can be complacency, procrastination, selective memory, and so on. Prejudices can mean how you feel about the older people, people with low income, or people of other races or religions.

Attitude 1: _____

Plan for improvement: _____

_____

Attitude 2: _____

Plan for improvement: _____

_____

The Language Barrier

Barriers in language that cause poor communication are called **semantic barriers**. These include using highly technical terms, abbreviations, and jargon. You should always try to be as specific as possible and leave no room for interpretation. For example: "I guess I should" would be better stated as, "I will." "Will one of you take care of this?" would be better stated as, "Juan, please take care of this."

Rewrite the following vague statements.

1. Do you think you could pick me up around 6?
    Improved communication: _____

2. Please make me a few copies.
    Improved communication: _____

3. Do you think you could try to lift this a couple of times?
    Improved communication: _____

4. I want only a few dollars for my old stethoscope.
    Improved communication: _____

5. I'm pretty sure you are doing better today.
    Improved communication: _____

Listening

Listening is the often forgotten communication tool. People tend to think of listening and **hearing** as the same thing. Nothing could be farther from the truth. We hear sounds with our ears, but we must listen with our brains. Listening implies paying attention and focusing on the sounds we hear. Listening requires us to concentrate and ignore all the other external and internal distractions. For example, external distractions can be found in a crowded room where we are trying to carry on a conversation. To truly listen, we must drown out all the extraneous noise and focus on the conversation we are part of. Internal distractions include our own mind going 100 miles an hour and not allowing us to focus on anything or anyone else.

Barriers to Effective Listening

Several barriers interfere with our ability to listen effectively. These, like communication barriers, include environmental and personal barriers. Environmental barriers include anything that can interfere with your ability to "hear" the message or any distractions that would interfere with your ability to focus. These include excessive noise levels, uncomfortable environmental conditions, and excessive visual stimulation. Personal barriers include physical and mental characteristics, preconceptions, and self-absorption.

Physical and Mental Characteristics. Listening is both a physical and mental activity. Without being able to hear properly, you lose your ability to effectively listen. The first prerequisite for effective listening is the ability to hear, and this should be assessed for any physiological impairments.

Mental characteristics can affect the ability to listen. If you are not "sharp and focused," your mind will tend to wander to other thoughts. Your physical body is present, but your mind is miles away. The term associated with this phenomenon is *daydreaming*. During long, one-sided conversations in which we are not actively involved in the communication process, we may find ourselves daydreaming.

Preconceptions. Have you ever listened to someone and thought, "They don't know what they are talking about"? You then have a *preconceived* idea that what this person has to say is useless, and therefore, you will not pay attention. This can be dangerous because then you are not open to other viewpoints that may differ from yours.

Self-Absorption. Have you ever politely listened to someone, while in your mind you were thinking about all the things you had to do? Sometimes we get so caught up in ourselves that it is hard to hear anyone else. This is called *self-absorption*.

Ways to Listen Effectively

One of the best methods for being an effective listener is to become an active listener as opposed to a passive listener. A passive listener pays just enough attention to keep the conversation going and appears interested. You can usually spot such people by their pleasant nods and frequent "uh-huhs." With these responses, the listener is trying to convince the speaker that they are paying attention.

Active listening is a must for important personal and professional communications. Active listening means that your mind is focused on both the message and the speaker. You are attempting to understand the verbal and nonverbal signals being sent your way.

One way to enhance active listening is to ask questions for clarification and to show that you have a curiosity and interest in the message. Another way to ensure that you listen actively is to take notes. Taking notes forces you to pay attention to the message and decide what is important enough to write down.

Another factor that enhances active listening is being open to other views that may conflict with yours. This does not mean that you agree with everything the speaker says but that you continue to actively listen and not "tune out" the message because you disagree with what it has to say.

Feedback is an important aspect to active listening and probably one of the most effective tools for improving communication. Requiring feedback concerning your message or giving feedback concerning someone else's message is crucial in ensuring that the message is clearly understood.

If you are delivering the message, the simplest way to gain feedback is to observe the receiver and judge the level of understanding. This can be done by looking for nonverbal cues, such as facial expressions. This form of feedback is possible only during face-to-face communication, when you can observe the receiver.

In any type of oral communication, whether it is face-to-face or otherwise, you can get feedback by asking questions or having the receiver repeat the information in their own words. Be careful that you ask questions that require more than just a yes or no response.

In general, the most effective questions are **open-ended questions**. Open-ended questions require an explanation as a response. Questions that begin with *what*, *how*, and *why* are generally open-ended questions. The questions "What do you think we have agreed on?" and "Why do you think you are getting this treatment?" are questions that require elaboration and can relate to you the receiver's level of understanding. **Close-ended questions** are those that can be answered with a simple yes or no. "Did you understand what I just said?" and "Are you feeling okay?" are examples of close-ended questions. To the first question, the feedback may be "yes," even though the patient did not fully understand what you were saying. The reason for this is that some patients may think that they will appear stupid if they say no. Patients may also say "yes" that they are feeling well, even though they are not because they are in denial and afraid to admit that something is wrong.

Finally, you can get feedback in a written format. For example, you may ask a patient to list the steps that you just explained for performing a procedure at home. This will tell you whether the patient really understands all the steps and the order in which they are to be done. Ways you can improve your listening skills include the following:

1. Avoid barriers such as furniture between you and the other person.
2. Get close to the other person but not so close that you invade the person's personal space and make them feel uncomfortable.
3. Sit at the patient's bedside when conversing, versus hovering over the patient, to make them feel comfortable.
4. Remain relaxed and friendly, and maintain good eye contact.
5. Do not be distracted by other unimportant events.
6. Have the patient paraphrase what was said to ensure understanding, and ask open-ended questions.
7. Be genuine and sincere. The patient will open up to you and feel more comfortable. The patient will be able to tell whether you are genuinely sincere or just faking interest.

Being a good listener can allow you to establish a positive relationship with your patient (Figure 7–3). Listening will also aid you in gaining valuable information that could assist in the diagnosis and treatment of the patient's condition.

Figure 7–3
Listen to your patients.

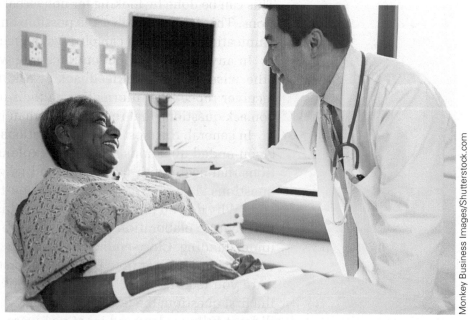

Monkey Business Images/Shutterstock.com

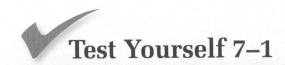

Test Yourself 7–1

How Well Do You Listen?

This is an assessment of your ability to listen effectively. Answer the following questions with this scale:

4 = Always   3 = Often   2 = Seldom   1 = Never

1. _____ I make eye contact with the speaker.

2. _____ I notice the speaker's nonverbal signals (body language).

3. _____ I allow the speaker to finish the complete thought without interruption.

4. _____ I have normal hearing.

5. _____ I ignore other sights and sounds when listening to someone speak.

6. _____ I concentrate on the speaker's thoughts and am not distracted by the way the message is delivered or by the person's appearance.

7. _____ I believe that by listening to other people I can always learn something.

8. _____ If I do not understand something, I ask the speaker to repeat it.

9. _____ I continue to listen even when I disagree with or am uncomfortable with what the speaker is saying.

10. _____ I do not pretend to be listening when I am really daydreaming or thinking about other things.

A score of 30 to 40 means that you are a good listener. A score of 20 to 30 means you can improve your listening skills, especially by focusing in on areas you rated as 1 and 2. A total of less than 20 means you are severely deficient in your listening ability and really need to work on this critical skill.

Skill Application 7–2 Environmental Barriers to Effective Listening

Listening is often neglected or considered to be a passive activity in the communication process. Nothing could be farther from the truth! Listening is one of the most active, dynamic, and effective tools in the communication process.

For one full day, take note of the environmental factors that can act as a barrier to effective listening. Give at least three examples, and explain how the environment can be improved.

Environmental barrier 1: _____

Environmental improvement: _____

_____

(continues)

(continued)

Environmental barrier 2: _____

Environmental improvement: _____

_____

Environmental barrier 3: _____

Environmental improvement: _____

_____

Personal Barriers to Effective Listening

Review the personal barriers for effective listening presented in this chapter. For one full day, take note of any of these personal barriers you observe in yourself or others. List three examples of personal barriers you have observed, and explain how they can be broken down.

Personal barrier 1: _____

Method to break down barrier: _____

_____

Personal barrier 2: _____

Method to break down barrier: _____

_____

Personal barrier 3: _____

Method to break down barrier: _____

_____

Feedback and Open-Ended Questions

List five open-ended questions you can ask your patient concerning the disease process or the effectiveness of treatment you will be providing.

Question 1: _____

Question 2: _____

Question 3: _____

Question 4: _____

Question 5: _____

Customer Relations

Customer relations refers to the way clients (patients and visitors) are treated by the employees of a business. Good customer relations are an essential ingredient in the success of any organization. It is especially important to health care because satisfied customers will return for more services and dissatisfied customers will quickly look elsewhere.

Good communications relate directly to good customer (patient) relations. Many times, choices are made on first impressions. This can often be on the first telephone call made to the health care facility. Proper telephone communication is a must for good customer relationships.

Many health care systems perform public outreach and service in the form of educational seminars and support groups. Therefore, it is important to possess good public speaking skills and understand how to effectively educate patients and their families.

Tips for Good Customer Relations

The following is a list of tips that will optimize good customer relations:

- Learn to recognize repeat customers' voices and identify them by name. Recognition means that you value their business.
- Listen carefully.
- Do not make customers repeat themselves. Take notes about the customer's problems or requests. This may include dates and times, order numbers, addresses, and other pertinent information.
- Think critically. You should consider what the customer tells you, eliminate unnecessary information, and pay attention to the heart of the problem or request.
- Do not interrupt. Sometimes customers feel better when they can talk things out. By interrupting, you may break their train of thought, miss crucial information, or increase the customer's anger and frustration.
- Ask questions to help clarify issues and information. Do not ask the same question repeatedly because this usually makes customers think you have not been listening to their responses.
- Solve problems and process requests according to company policy.

- Keep your word. If you say you will call back or take some other action, do it in a timely manner.
- Before terminating a telephone call or personal encounter, ask if there is anything else the person wishes to discuss or if any additional help is needed.
- Follow up. Check with the client later to ensure that everything was done satisfactorily; this shows you value their patronage.

Telephone Etiquette

Your first contact and impression about many organizations occur over the telephone. As has been discussed, you never get a second chance to make a good first impression. Companies realize the importance of good **telephone etiquette** as it relates to favorable customer impressions and satisfaction.

When speaking on the telephone, unless Facetiming, you lose the nonverbal feedback that is so valuable in effective communications. Therefore, you must compensate for the lack of being able to read someone's facial expressions or body language. You must focus on your choice of words and voice quality to effectively communicate your message.

Here are some hints on proper telephone use:

- Greeting: Immediately identify yourself and your company or department. For example, "Hello, this is Jane Smith from the radiology department at Acme Hospital. How can I help you?"
- Voice: Talk directly into the mouthpiece, about an inch away, to ensure clarity. Do not eat or drink while talking on the telephone. The annoying sounds can be heard on the other end. Speak in a clear and normal volume, and pay particular attention to enunciation. Remember to vary your tone, pitch, and volume for emphasis and to maintain interest.
- Use common courtesy: Be friendly and *smile*; this will come through in your voice (Figure 7–4). Use the other person's name in your conversation and do not interrupt. If you need to place someone on hold, explain that you will be right back. Be polite. Saying *please* and *thank you* show courtesy, and courtesy shows respect for the caller. If using a landline, when you hang up, gently place the receiver back on the hook; the other person may still be on the line.
- Pay attention: This shows interest. Picture the person on the other end of the telephone, and focus on what is being said.

Always remember that your behavior on the telephone represents the company as well as your personality. How well your company does relates to job security and the potential for your advancement.

Figure 7–4
Your attitude comes
through on the telephone.

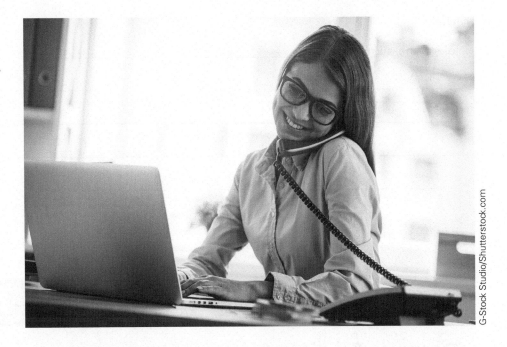

G-Stock Studio/Shutterstock.com

Skill Application 7–3 Appreciation of Customer Relations

Good customer relations are crucial for the success of any organization.

1. Pick an organization that you have had recent positive contact with and list three areas of customer relations that impressed you.

   a. _____

   b. _____

   c. _____

2. List three customer relations tips you think would be essential for health care practitioners to use on a daily basis.

   a. _____

   b. _____

   c. _____

Answering the Telephone

The telephone is often the first contact a customer has with an organization. Each company should have a protocol for answering the telephone. Develop a telephone etiquette policy for a health care department within a hospital. This policy should include protocol for how to handle incoming calls, what to include in the initial greeting, how to take and deliver messages, and who is to handle specific types of calls (e.g., complaints, billing). For example, a part of the policy for the greeting could state that you identify the department, yourself, and your title and then ask, "May I help you?"

(continues)

(continued)

Telephone etiquette policy: _____

_____

_____

_____

Food **for** Thought 7–2

Customer Relations Assessment

Assess an organization you have had recent contact with in light of the previous reading on customer relations.

1. List three things they did well and give specific examples.

   a. _____

   b. _____

   c. _____

2. List three areas that need improvement and provide specific examples of how their customer relations can be improved.

   a. _____

   b. _____

   c. _____

3. Finally, how does good customer relations "relate" to individual job security?

_____

_____

_____

Technological Communication

While face-to-face communication may be the mode of choice in most health care situations, technological communication is also prevalent. Technological communication methods can include fax machines, e-mails, teleconferencing, and text messaging via cell phones. The basic principles of good communication still hold true. Keep the message simple and direct. However, there are some considerations that must be kept in mind as you are composing your electronic message. In most cases, the receiver will not see facial expressions or hear different vocal inflections that may convey added meaning. Therefore, attempt to keep your message as clear as possible and not open to many interpretations. In addition, you must make sure that the message has been properly sent and received because many things can go wrong in cyberspace.

E-mail is a popular and effective mode of electronic communication because it is:

- Less expensive than mailing a letter
- Usually much faster than the postal service (hence, the term "snail mail" is given to postal mail)
- More conversational in nature
- Less intrusive than a telephone call or fax
- Can readily reach targeted groups of individuals

However, it is not without problems. You should keep in mind the following important points concerning e-mail communication:

- Make sure that your subject line clearly states the content of the message, or it may be filtered as junk mail and never reach your intended receiver.
- Double-check your addressee because one misplaced letter can send it to the wrong person.
- Be VERY careful when hitting the reply button if the message was sent to a group of people. There have been many cases where a reply was meant only for the sender's eyes but was sent back to the entire group.
- Do not use e-mail jargon that you use with your friends, and be sure to spell out each word and use correct grammar and punctuation.
- You should never send protected health information (PHI) via e-mail; it can easily end up in the wrong hands. Many health care facilities require a disclaimer go at the bottom of the e-mail, telling the receiver what to do in case they get an e-mail that does not belong to them.

Web pages are a very important way an organization can market itself and allow for contact with potential clients. In addition to the jazzy graphics and pictures, websites should contain clear and concise information, be easy to navigate, and have contact information such as phone numbers, e-mail addresses, and directions on how to find the organization.

Public Speaking

Health care practitioners are often called on to speak to groups of people. These presentations can be informal or formal in nature and can be presented to patients, families, community groups, or other health care professionals.

The three most important rules for an effective presentation are to (1) be prepared, (2) be prepared, and (3) be prepared. Know your subject area well, and organize your presentation in a logical manner that makes sense and is easy to follow. After you have researched your topic well, ask yourself the following questions:

- Who is my audience, and how can I best relate to them?
- What is my audience's interest in the subject?
- Is a formal or informal presentation best?
- What type of supporting materials (handouts) would be beneficial?
- What type of audiovisual material will be most effective for this group?

Think about what type of presenters stimulated your interest most. It was probably people whom you could relate to. It is important to be yourself and let the audience see who you are. Facts and figures are important, but you need to make them relevant to your audience while not overwhelming them.

Preparing a simple and logical outline for yourself and your audience will help keep you focused and organized. Keep in mind that there are three important parts to your presentation: the introduction, body, and conclusion.

Make sure you have a good *introduction* that catches attention, draws your audience in, and shows the relevance of your talk. Practice the introduction so it looks natural because people pay most attention at the beginning and that sets the tone for how engaged they will stay throughout your presentation.

Next work on the body of your presentation. Remember, people have a difficult time with too much information at once, so keep the *body* of the presentation simple. Three or four main points are all you need. If you have definitions or graphs, include them on a note-taking outline so that the audience can spend less time writing feverishly and more time listening to what you have to say.

Finally, it is very important to have a strong *conclusion!* This again should be practiced so it appears natural. Your introduction drew the audience in and now your conclusion will leave a powerful lasting impression.

Food **for** Thought 7–3

Learn from Others

Think about a favorite teacher or a presentation you attended. What are five characteristics that made a favorable impression on you?

Patient Communication and Education

Communicating with patients is crucial for effective assessment, diagnosis, and treatment. Remember, you are there to provide care and support to the patient. Be open, supportive, and courteous in all your interactions. The following are factors to consider for effective patient interaction.

- Answer call bells promptly.
- Focus on the patient's need(s).
- Make sure that you have the patient's attention.
- Speak clearly, using a pleasant tone.
- Use appropriate body language that indicates your interest and concern. Touch the patient, if it seems appropriate. Lean forward, listen to what the patient is saying verbally and nonverbally, and maintain eye contact.
- Allow time for the patient to ask questions.
- Evaluate the patient's verbal and nonverbal responses to assess understanding or treatment effectiveness.
- Ask for feedback in the form of open-ended questions and return demonstrations of procedures.
- Use visual aids if possible.
- Use good listening techniques.

Always include family members when possible, in patient education. If a technique is being taught, make sure you request a return demonstration by the patient to make sure they understand and are performing correctly all the steps. Make sure the patient understands their medications, how and when to take, how to get refills, and what side effects can occur.

Skill Application 7–4 Patient Education

Public speaking plays an important role in effective patient education. Develop a 20-minute presentation to a group of patients on one of the following topics:

A group of children, aged 7 to 10 years, on the disease and treatment of asthma

A group of patients with heart disease concerning proper nutrition and exercise

A group of patients with allergies on how to assess and treat the home environment to minimize respiratory problems

A group of patients with diabetes concerning proper understanding and treatment of their disease

Note: Include objectives, outline, handouts, and method of evaluating the level of understanding of the material you presented.

Recording and Reporting Information

In health care, an important part of communication is observing or assessing a patient and then recording and reporting this information. You will have to use your sense of sight to observe the patient for color changes, indications of pain, physical abnormalities, levels of distress, and so on. Your sense of smell will help you identify odors that could alert you to certain types of infections. Your sense of touch is critical in feeling for (palpating) a pulse, noting skin warmth, assessing swelling (edema), and performing many therapeutic techniques. Your sense of hearing is needed for listening to the lungs (auscultation), taking a blood pressure, and hearing other normal and abnormal body sounds. Hearing is also needed for effective listening to occur when taking a patient history and identifying the chief complaint. By using all your senses, you can gain a lot of information concerning your patient's condition. The next step is to now record that information properly in the health record and also to give a verbal report (hand off) to the appropriate persons so the information

Figure 7–5
Recording and reporting patient information is crucial.

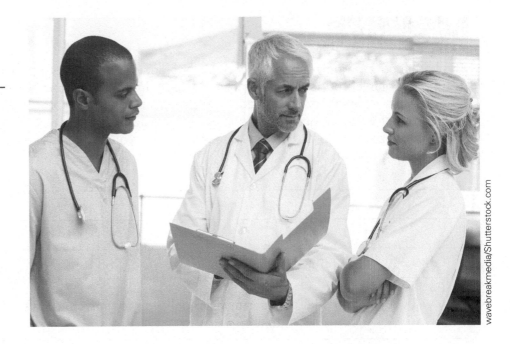

wavebreakmedia/Shutterstock.com

is correctly passed on (Figure 7–5). Charting and giving reports are covered in an upcoming chapter. For now, just realize it is also an important part of the communication process in giving high-quality care to patients.

Summary

- For communication to truly be effective, you must assess and remove the environmental and personal factors that can impair the communication process.

- Environmental or physical barriers can include noise, activity levels, room arrangement, comfort levels, technological problems, and time or distance issues.

- Personal barriers include emotions, attitudes, prejudices, complacency, and language issues.

- An often forgotten part of the communication process is listening. Again, you must break down the barriers that inhibit listening and learn to become an active listener.

- In a health care organization, patients, families, and visitors all represent customers. Therefore, good customer relation skills must be practiced.

- Technological communication and reporting skills are prevalent in all areas of health care, and therefore, your skills in these areas need to be maximized.

- Health care practitioners are often needed to do public and patient education and need to enhance their public speaking skills.

Case Study 7–1

The health care organization you work for has decided to do more public education programs. You have volunteered to do a program on teaching children and their parents how to better manage their asthma. Your organization feels that a high-quality program will attract more clients and can, therefore, be greatly beneficial to the organization's health. This could mean a future promotion for your efforts. List three specific actions you can take to ensure that this is indeed a high-quality program.

_____

_____

_____

_____

How will you need to adjust the communication levels for this program?

_____

_____

How will you obtain feedback to assess the effectiveness of your program?

_____

_____

Internet Activity

Using Internet search engines, find additional material on "communication in action" that can help you and your fellow students. Some suggested keywords are active listening, telephone etiquette, customer relations, communication barriers, and public speaking. Write down something new that you found to share.

_____

_____

_____

Chapter 8

Communication within an Organization

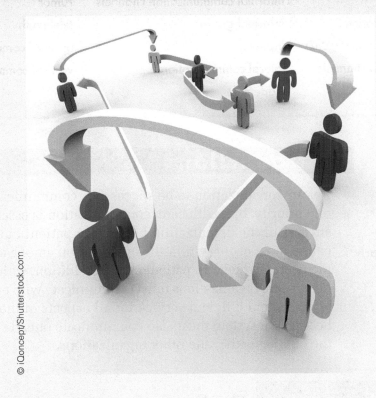

© iQoncept/Shutterstock.com

Objectives

Upon completion of this chapter, you should be able to:

1. Describe the health care system.

2. Describe organizational structure, communication channels, and lines of authority.

3. Define the factors that affect group dynamics.

4. Demonstrate optimal group interaction skills.

5. Utilize group interaction skills to maximize your leadership potential.

6. Identify ways to succeed in the clinical learning environment.

7. Define cultural competency.

Key Terms

cohesiveness	gossip	line of authority
conformity	group dynamics	norms
cultural competency	groupthink	organizational chart
diagonal communication	horizontal communication	outpatient
dialysis	informal communication channels	rumor
downward communication	informal group	telehealth
durable medical equipment (DME)	inpatient	upward communication
formal communication channels	lateral communication	vertical communication
formal group	leadership	

Introduction

The nice thing about teamwork is that you always have others on your side.

—Margaret Carty

For any organization to be successful, communication is the number one priority. In health care, communication is essential not just to the success of the organization but also to patient outcomes. Communication must occur within the organization among all health care team members involved in patient care. In addition, various departments in health care organizations must communicate with each other to deliver effective and efficient service for all aspects of the organization. The health care system must also communicate outside the organization to the public, media, and other organizations.

Anticipatory Exercise 8–1   The Gossip Game

The grapevine can be a powerful communication tool in the organization. However, it can often distort, exaggerate, or disrupt the communication of the organization. See if the following exercise demonstrates this concept.

1. Form a group of at least 10 individuals. Designate one individual to make up a fictitious story concerning an organization. The story should be at least one typewritten double-spaced page.

2. Form a circle and have this individual whisper the story (reading it exactly as written) into the ear of the person seated next to them.

3. Allow the story to be passed on (whispered) to each individual in the circle. Have the last person who receives the story stand up and recite their version of the story out loud to the entire group.

4. Finally, have the first individual read the story from the page and compare the results.

Briefly describe the results of this exercise and what it demonstrated to you. _____

_____

_____

_____

The Health Care System: An Overview

Health care delivery in the United States is an extremely large and complex system. It is beyond the scope of this text to go into detail, but a brief overview is provided. Hospitals are the largest employers and are still the main resource for health care in the United States. With rising costs and advancements in technology, we have seen a decrease in the number of days that a patient stays in a hospital. A person who stays overnight or for more than 1 day is known as an **inpatient**. The hospital's focus is now more on the type of individual who comes in for a procedure and leaves the same day. As a result, we are seeing more emphasis on **outpatient** care.

There are a variety of ways that hospitals can be classified. We can have rural or community hospitals. *General hospitals* provide routine care and specialized care such as emergency departments and intensive care units. *Teaching hospitals* are similar to general hospitals but are usually located near a medical school. As a result, medical students, interns, and residents treat patients under the supervision of the hospital's staff physicians. In a teaching hospital, there may be a greater variety of specialists on staff to train the interns and residents. *Research hospitals* provide patient care and also conduct research on the causes, prevention, and treatment of disease. Hospitals can be classified by their *specialty* such as pediatric hospitals, women's hospitals, burn hospitals, orthopedic hospitals, or cancer hospitals. Often, hospitals are classified as *governmental* or *nongovernmental*. Examples of governmental hospitals would be Veterans Administration hospitals, military hospitals, and Indian Health Service hospitals.

There are free standing ambulatory surgical centers or outpatient surgical facilities where people can have procedures done such as cataract removal, tonsillectomy, or other minor procedures. It is often more cost effective than having a procedure in a hospital.

There are free standing birth centers that focus on childbirth. They are often home-like environments that are comfortable for the person laboring. These facilities must have an arrangement with a nearby hospital in case of emergency.

Dialysis centers are places where people who need **dialysis** (a process that cleans and filters the blood when the kidneys no longer work) can receive treatment. Most people on dialysis need treatments three times a week, and they can take up to 4 hours to complete. It is estimated that 14% of the U.S. population gets dialysis. Often there is a need for a facility that provides urgent, but not emergency, care when a physician's office is closed or an individual is not near their physician's office. The *urgent care center* has been created to meet this need. These facilities can treat infections, draw blood for testing, conduct physicals, and complete basic diagnostics. Usually there is quick patient assessment with little waiting. As a result, workers' compensation cases and occupational medicine coverage because of workplace injuries can be performed here for companies. Often these centers are designated as primary care facilities for various managed care systems.

Long-term care institutions have been created for individuals who are too weak or sick to care for themselves in a home setting. While many long-term care institutions are owned and operated by various church groups, the bulk of them are owned and run by health care corporations for profit. It is estimated that approximately 8% of the U.S. population over 65 years of age (roughly 1.2 million people) are residents in long-term care facilities. In recent years, regulations and quality standards have been raised for these types of institutions. As a result, the cost to the consumer has also increased, forcing many patients to utilize Medicaid (a national form of health insurance for the people with low income) once they use up all of their personal funds.

There are three main classifications of long-term care institutions:

- *Skilled nursing facilities* (SNFs)
- *Intermediate care facilities* (ICFs)
- *Extended care facilities* (ECFs)

Skilled nursing facilities are for individuals who need around-the-clock skilled nursing care such as long-term mechanical ventilator support. Currently, patients in SNFs are required to be recertified every 100 days to allow them to maintain residence in these types of facilities. *Intermediate care facilities* are for individuals who would no longer have the capability to live alone and care for themselves but do not need around-the-clock skilled nursing care. Rehabilitative and occupational therapists are often available for the patients in this type of facility to help them with activities of daily living. If a patient no longer needs skilled nursing care and is still either too incapacitated or ill to live at home, they may reside in an *extended care facility*. In this scenario, custodial care is provided for the patient to provide minimal assistance with their activities of daily living.

An *assisted living facility* provides a living situation for an older adult or couple who can take care of themselves with minimum supervision. In this case, an apartment is utilized for a fixed fee with some meals and services provided.

Rehabilitation hospitals can be free standing or on a floor or wing of a hospital. A patient must be able to participate in 3 hours of therapy per day to qualify for admission. These facilities cater to patients who have had orthopedic surgery or are recovering from trauma such as a motor vehicle accident.

Mental health and addiction treatment centers exist in many different forms. Some are free standing, some are day programs, and others are part of a hospital. They can treat mental health issues such as depression, eating disorders, or substance abuse disorders.

Telehealth is one of the most rapidly growing ways to deliver health care. Telehealth use became widespread during the COVID-19 pandemic and is now mainstream. Telehealth involves the use of electronic communication between the provider and the patient. This is usually done via a secure meeting platform often incorporated into an electronic health record on the provider end; the patient can use any device such as a personal computer, laptop, or smartphone.

Home health agencies may or may not be affiliated with a hospital. Home health agencies provide care for a patient in their home. They may provide homemaker services (cooking, cleaning, and meal preparation) or intermittent skilled care. Some agencies provide around-the-clock nursing care to qualifying patients.

When most people hear the term *hospice*, they immediately think of a building where people go to die. Hospice is an interdisciplinary program that provides end-of-life support for the terminally ill patient, the family, and/or significant others. While the terminal disease is not actively being treated, supportive (palliative) care, such as pain management, is provided. Other services that address additional physical, emotional, spiritual, economic, and social needs are provided. Most hospice care occurs in the home, although there are also hospice centers where patients can go.

Durable medical equipment (DME) suppliers provide patients with the adaptive equipment they may need to live at home. This may be respiratory supplies (home oxygen or ventilators), walkers, wheelchairs, or prosthetics to name a few. Some DME companies also provide pharmaceuticals supplies such as wound dressings. Many DME companies employ health care providers to educate and set up the equipment.

Clinical laboratories can be within a hospital or stand alone. This is where a person can go to have blood tests drawn and other tests like urine drug screens.

Ambulance companies provide emergency responses along with scheduled transport for people who are unable to ride in a car to appointments. Reasons a person cannot take a car include dependence on a ventilator or needing a special lift to transfer from bed to chair.

As you can see, good communication is vital to all health care facilities, regardless of the setting not only for the health care team but also for the patients, family members, and loved ones.

Food **for** Thought 8–1

Legislation and Health Care

The main characteristics that define the U.S. health care systems are the lack of a central governing agency, the focus on acute care, the expense, and the unequal access based on insurance coverage. The Affordable Care Act passed in 2010 is the U.S. government's attempt to decrease health care cost and provide insurance coverage to all Americans. This law has faced much debate, and it has been upheld by the Supreme Court and is in effect. More information on the Affordable Care Act can be found at https://www.hhs.gov/healthcare/index.html.

Communication Networks

To help employees understand how the organization is put together, an **organizational chart** is developed. This chart succinctly shows many characteristics concerning the organization. The chart shows the flow of communication, the relationships among various departments, and the lines of authority. Figure 8–1 shows a portion of a health care system's organizational chart.

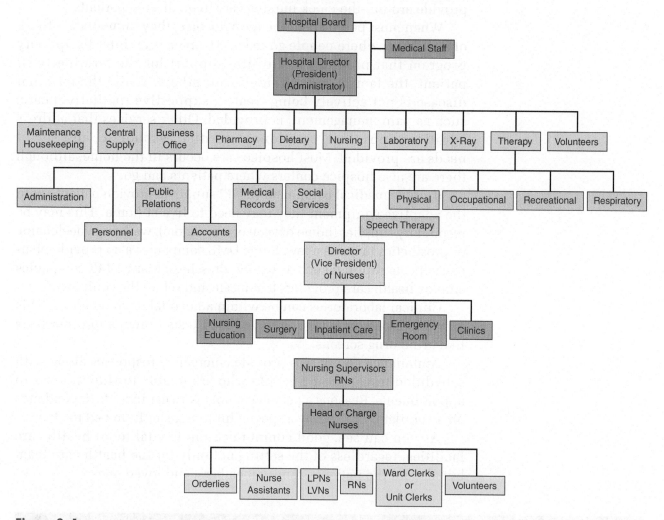

Figure 8–1
An example of a health care organizational chart.

Food **for** Thought 8–2

The Proper Channels

You probably have heard the expression "make sure you go through the proper channels." What does this mean to you? What are the formal channels of communication within your school? What are the informal channels of communication?

In addition to the organizational chart, every organization has two separate communication channels broken down along formal and informal lines. **Formal communication channels** are established by the way the organization is put together. You can see much of the flow of communication by viewing an organizational structure or flowchart. The **informal communication channels** are sometimes referred to as the "grapevine." Each channel is very powerful and can have a positive or negative effect on the organization's functioning. Formal and informal channels relay messages from one person or group to another in a downward, upward, horizontal, or diagonal direction.

Directions of Communication Flow

Information can flow through an organization in a variety of directions. **Downward communication** is a formal flow of communication from people with formal power (managers or supervisors) to staff employees. The flow begins with someone at the top of the structure communicating a message to the next person or group within the hierarchy. This person or persons will then pass it along to those within their group and downward if needed.

Upward communication comes from the staff employees and flows upward to the person or persons in charge. This is as important as downward communication. Be careful not to attach levels of importance to communication channels. All communication is critical, whether it be a directive issued downward from management or a serious problem identified by a staff employee that needs to be brought to a supervisor's attention through upward communication. The supervisor must keep the staff informed, and the employees must feel free to convey opinions and attitudes and to report on the activities of their work.

The combination of upward and downward communication is sometimes called **vertical communication**. Some typical examples of vertical communication are as follows:

- Policies from the management
- Finished products and reports from the staff
- Supervisors' communication with the staff
- Staff communication upward to supervisors
- Written memos, e-mails, letters, and formal reports
- Formal meetings or training sessions

Horizontal communication, or **lateral communication**, is mainly used when departments or groups of people on the same level of the organizational chart need to talk with each other. These may be two departments that are in charge of two different areas where activities overlap. For example, lateral communication often occurs between a nursing floor and the radiological department to schedule procedures. This is important because patients have several other procedures that

Figure 8–2
Lines of authority.

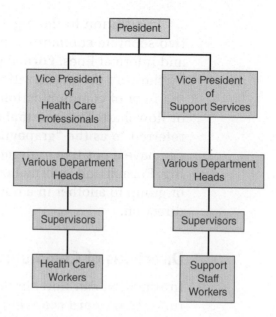

need to be done, and therefore, the nursing department needs to know when to deliver the patient, how long the test will take, and whether there are any special precautions or diets that need to be observed before the test. Horizontal communication is important in facilitating coordination.

Diagonal communication is the flow of communication between departments or people that are on different lateral planes of the organizational chart. For example, nursing personnel may need to contact the housekeeping department when a patient leaves so that the room can be readied for the next patient. To achieve optimal efficiency, effectiveness, and coordination among the various elements of any organization—especially in a health care organization—a free flow of all types of communication (upward, downward, diagonal, and horizontal) is essential.

Someone always has to be in a position to make the final decision or to decide what message is to be sent. The **line of authority** begins at the top of the organizational chart and can be traced downward throughout the entire organization (Figure 8–2). The line of authority defines the chain of command and establishes the flow of information and responsibility from one individual to another and between departments.

The Grapevine: The Informal Channel of Communication

There was a popular song in the 1960s called "I Heard It through the Grapevine." Unfortunately, as the song illustrates, this is not the best way to hear information. The grapevine may or may not contain factual information. Often, the information contained in the grapevine is based on rumor or gossip. **Rumor** refers to information presented as fact but which has not been officially confirmed. An example of a rumor may be the downsizing of a certain department or division.

Gossip is more personal in nature and is usually directed at an individual or group of individuals. Some of the characteristics of the grapevine that often make it an undesirable route of communication are as follows:

- Information may be incomplete.
- Information may be based on rumor or gossip and not on facts.
- Information may be distorted or exaggerated as it is repeatedly passed on.
- Information may include emotional and prejudicial statements caused by each person's personal feelings.

One way to not become entangled in the grapevine is to avoid office gossip. This will make you stand out as someone who can be trusted with confidential information. Keep what you hear through the grapevine to yourself and do not spread gossip. Stand up for your coworkers when others make unsubstantiated statements about them. This will increase your status within a department as an individual with integrity and one who can be trusted.

Food for Thought 8–3

The Office Gossip

You probably know people who gossip a lot. How do you feel about them? Can you trust them with information? Can they maintain confidentiality in the health care setting? Why do people gossip at the office? Have you ever heard of management using the grapevine to disseminate information (especially bad news)?

Skill Application 8–1 The Organizational Chart

Pick an organization that you are involved with and obtain and draw its organizational chart. If the chart is extensive, pick a portion that will fit onto this page. You can use your school.

Understanding the Organizational Chart

Understanding the lines of communication within an organization is essential to your success within the organization.

1. From the chart you have drawn, give a description of the informational channels that exist.

   _____

   _____

   _____

   _____

(continues)

(continued)

2. Now, identify the following on your chart and briefly describe each:

Vertical communication channels: _____

_____

_____

Horizontal communication channels: _____

_____

_____

Diagonal communication channels: _____

_____

_____

Working within a Group

No matter where you work (unless you isolate yourself from society), you will need to understand how to effectively function within a group. Groups can be either formal or informal in nature. A **formal group** is a collection of people who share clear goals and expectations along with established rules of conduct. As a health care practitioner, your coworkers within your department would represent a formal group of individuals. They would share the common goals associated with quality patient care and the efficient running of the department.

An **informal group** is a loose association of people without stated rules or goals. A group of people at a party or waiting in line for a movie would represent an informal group. Although there are no stated rules in an informal group, there are certain unwritten rules of behavior that are dictated by societal values. For example, skipping ahead in line or starting a fight at a party would be unacceptable behaviors. All groups, whether formal or informal, share certain standards of behavior and characteristic communication patterns that are unique to the group. In other words, people behave differently in groups than they do individually. Understanding these differences will make you an effective group member and enable you to develop team skills that will help you in all areas of your life.

Group Dynamics

Group dynamics is the study of how people interact in groups. This includes group goals, individual roles, communication patterns, and factors that enhance cohesiveness and positive group interaction. We will now take a more in-depth look at each of these factors.

Group Goals

Just as goals are important for the individual, they are also critical for groups in order to bring focus and direction. Ideally, goals should be developed and agreed on by the group. Just like individual goals, they should be positive and measurable.

Group goals can be cooperative or competitive in nature. Goals are cooperative when the people work together to achieve an objective. A sports team working together to win a game is an example of a cooperative goal. However, competitive goals also exist within the team. For example, each member may be committed to winning as a team but may also have a competitive goal of being the best to get more playing time or to have greater individual recognition.

Most groups have both cooperative and competitive goals. Health care systems in today's environment are organizing their workers into teams or task forces. Members of the team must cooperate with one another to achieve the goals of the team while at the same time possibly competing with other teams in the organization or other outside competitors. Within the team, cooperative goals must be the focus because they enhance communication and productivity. If competitive goals become the major focus, there can be rivalries and secretiveness, which can inhibit communication. However, competitive goals can be a positive stimulus when they create feelings of challenge and excitement and motivate people to do their best.

Individual Roles

Each person on a team or within a group has a set of expected behavior or responsibilities. These define the individual roles within the group. Roles state what you are expected to do. Within groups, there are certain expectations, or **norms**, by which people in particular roles are expected to adhere.

For example, your role within a health care department may be as a shift supervisor. This job role defines your expected behavior for that position. You may be expected to dole out the work, evaluate employees, mediate conflict, order supplies, and so on. The norms for this position would be someone who is dependable, is hard working, and has good interpersonal and organizational skills.

In many formal groups, specific roles are assigned to members. For example, a professional organization that represents your chosen health career may have a president, vice president, secretary, and treasurer. In addition, there may be several committees concerning patient care, legislation, communication, membership, and so on. Each committee may have a chairperson whose function is to schedule and run the meeting. A recording secretary may be responsible for recording and distributing the minutes.

Communication Patterns

Communication within groups can take on various patterns (Figure 8–3). For example, a formal group may have a rigid chain of command that dictates that messages are to be passed down from the top of the organization to the bottom. This can be represented as a chain pattern of communication. Notice how only the links that interconnect are in direct communication.

Another example of a formal communication pattern is called the wheel pattern. Here, one person is the central distributor and controller of the informational flow. An example of this type may be a health care office manager who directs the front desk, billing, nurses, and therapists.

In most organizations, open communication with all members is encouraged. Even in large organizations, tasks and strategic planning are done in smaller, less formal groups known as project teams

Figure 8–3
Various communication patterns of groups.

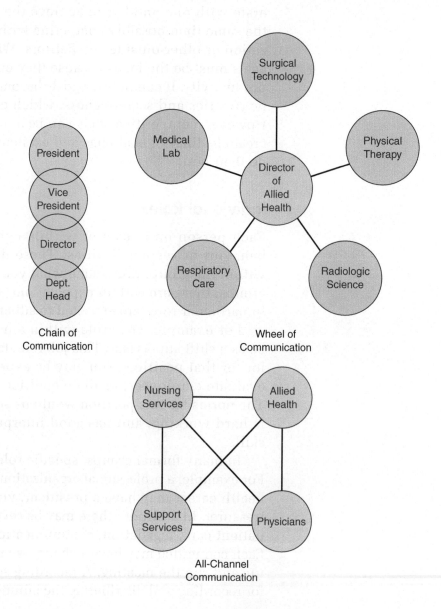

Chain of
Communication

Wheel of
Communication

All-Channel
Communication

or focused task groups. Here all group members are free to communicate with one another in an open or all-channel pattern of communication. Again, see Figure 8–3, which depicts various group communication patterns.

Cohesiveness

All groups have various levels of **cohesiveness**. Cohesiveness is measured by the degree to which members work together. Highly cohesive groups tend to have clearly defined roles and goals to which they are strongly committed. Pride and loyalty run high in these groups. Low-cohesive groups tend to be very vague about their goals, and members do not know what is expected of them. Low commitment and motivation characterize low-cohesive groups.

Group Interaction

Several different interactions that can occur within a group do not tend to occur with individual communications. One such phenomenon deals with group conformity. Changing your opinion or behavior in response to pressure from a group is called **conformity**. Have you ever found yourself doing something just because everyone else is doing it? You may have even done something that went against your personal values or beliefs because you wanted to be accepted as part of the group. It can be very dangerous when an individual gives up their values and beliefs and does what the group is doing regardless of the consequences.

Psychologists believe that people who conform to group behavior that is contrary to their beliefs and values have low self-esteem and confidence. In essence, if you conform to the group against your beliefs, the group is thinking for you and deciding what is right and wrong. It is important to act independently when group values contradict your own values.

Conformity is not always a bad thing. In common social group situations, such as a classroom, we conform to the standards by not being disruptive to the educational process. Within a hospital, we conform to the standards of appropriate behavior. For example, a loud and verbally abusive employee is not conforming to the standards of behavior. Here, conformity is good. Remember to be aware when group norms go against your individual values. The important thing about conformity is to know when it is appropriate. Conformity carried to the extreme can lead to **groupthink**. Groupthink is the unquestioning acceptance of the group's beliefs and behaviors. The group becomes the only voice determining what or who is right and wrong. Loyalty to the group becomes more important than anything else. This is a dangerous situation that causes members to lose their ability to think critically and independently. They also compromise their individual values and beliefs. Groups experiencing extreme groupthink can become paranoid and develop an "us against them attitude."

Food **for** Thought 8–4

Groupthink

Can you think of situations in which conformity can be dangerous? What about situations when conformity is appropriate? Can you describe how groupthink can lead to prejudices, hatred, and even wars? Can you give a historical example?

Skill Application 8–2 Types of Groups

The understanding of the group process is an important first step in maximizing your ability to work effectively within a team or group of people. Answer the following questions concerning the group process.

1. Identify a formal group that you are a member of. _____

2. List the goals of this group. _____

    _____

3. Elaborate on your specific role within this group. _____

    _____

4. What type of communication pattern exists? _____

5. How would you characterize the group cohesiveness? _____

    _____

6. List factors that are detrimental to group cohesiveness. _____

    _____

    _____

7. List factors that enhance group cohesiveness. _____

    _____

    _____

8. Give two examples of informal groups. _____

    _____

(continues)

(continued)

Conformity and Groupthink

1. Give an example of when conformity to group norms can be dangerous or simply wrong. _____
   _____
   _____

2. Give an example of when conformity to group norms is acceptable. _____
   _____
   _____

3. Elaborate on an example of when a group is experiencing groupthink. Either use a group you are personally familiar with or use a group of people from history. _____
   _____
   _____
   _____

4. List the negative outcomes of groupthink to both the group and people outside the group. _____
   _____
   _____
   _____

Effective Group Participation

You can use your knowledge of individual communication techniques coupled with your knowledge about how groups work to optimize your interaction with others. One of the first tasks you should undertake when joining any group is assessment. Group assessment should include understanding and defining group goals and norms. In addition, you should develop a clear understanding of your role within the group. Common questions you should be able to answer for effective group assessment include the following:

- What are the goals of the group?
- Are the group's goals cooperative or competitive (or both)?
- What pattern of communication exists?
- Is this a formal, semiformal, or informal group?
- What is my role within this group?

- What are the other members' roles?
- Does the group have a leader? Who is the leader?
- What are the group norms?

Having assessed the group, your next step is becoming an active participant in the group process. The answers to the preceding questions will help guide your behavior so that you become an accepted, functioning member of the group. For example, if this is a formal group with a set agenda and defined rules of order, you must act in that manner. However, if this is an informal group, you can be more casual in your behavior.

Being prepared for the discussion at hand is very important and demonstrates your interest and research capabilities. If you know the agenda or items to be discussed beforehand, you should be prepared to discuss these subjects intelligently. Preparation should include thinking about the subject and reading any relevant or related information.

Using your listening skills will help you become an informed member of the group. Pay attention and keep focused on the subject being discussed. It is beneficial in many situations to take notes, especially if an assignment and deadline are given.

Actively participate by sharing your ideas and respecting the ideas of others, even if you do not agree with them. Be courteous and cooperative with your fellow group members. Take pride in the group and your ability to enhance its functioning.

Group Leadership

Groups need all levels of participants to function effectively, but often a leader is chosen or naturally emerges from within a group. Sometimes the leadership of the group is rotated so that everyone gets a chance. Therefore, it is important that you understand the necessary skills required to lead a group.

Leadership is more than a position or title; it is an attitude and presence. Leadership is a set of behaviors, attitudes, and values that enables the leader to motivate and direct others to act. No matter what is written about leadership techniques, *the most effective still is leadership by example.*

It is, therefore, important to develop those qualities that will distinguish you as a leader. Although some people's magnetic or charismatic personalities may make them "born to lead," all of us can learn to become good leaders, even without natural charisma. Most people look for "ordinary but consistent" qualities in a leader that allow them to respect and trust the leader. Qualities such as the ability to get along with others, good communication skills, trustworthiness, and a strong commitment to goals will make others view you as a potential leader.

Skill Application 8–3 Group Assessment

Assess a formal group in which you are a member by answering the following questions:

1. Are the group goals cooperative, competitive, or a mix of both? _____

2. Is the communication formal or casual? _____

3. What are the various roles within this group? _____

   _____

4. What are the group norms? _____

   _____

   _____

5. Who is the group leader? _____

6. How can I maximize my potential within this group? _____

   _____

Group Leadership

1. From your previous group assessment, list the skills needed to become an effective leader within your group. _____

   _____

2. Which of these skills do you already possess? _____

   _____

3. What skills do you need to improve? _____

   _____

4. How can you improve your leadership skills? _____

   _____

Brainstorming

Another group technique an organization can use to foster creative thinking and generate ideas is brainstorming. Although the term *brainstorming* was coined in the 1950s and has been called several things since, *brainstorming* still says it the best. Group brainstorming is defined as providing an atmosphere in which ideas about any topic, problem, or opportunity can be freely generated. Brainstorming has received attention in business and industry, with much research generated on this process. The literature shows that there are some important criteria for this process to be maximally effective. These include the following:

- No judgment or evaluation should be made until all the ideas are presented.
- The quantity and *not* the quality of ideas is the major goal.
- Encourage unusual ideas and piggybacking on others' ideas.
- Choose an effective group leader to direct the process.
- Optimal group size is five to eight people.

Brainstorming, when done right, promotes progressive employee attitudes that help develop a sense of teamwork and camaraderie. This process helps unclog the communication channels and provides greater mutual respect between individuals and departments.

It is important to do this process right or it can create problems. Some of the pitfalls to avoid in the brainstorming process include a lack of understanding of the brainstorming process and the over-selling of the benefits. It will not cure all your problems, but it will generate ideas and increase group cohesiveness if everyone feels free to contribute.

A group leader who can present the problem or opportunity in a positive manner is critical. The leader must not allow any premature criticism, even something as subtle as someone rolling one's eyes. The leader must encourage everyone to contribute. In addition, adequate time should be given for the process to take place. The leader should also provide feedback and praise to the participants and follow up with the results of any of the ideas that may have been implemented as a result of the brainstorming process. Brainstorming can be fun, energizing, motivating, and highly productive if done correctly. However, if done improperly, it can be perceived as a waste of time by the participants. Refer to Chapter 4 for a detailed discussion of brainstorming.

✔ Test Yourself 8–1

Leadership Skills

Rate yourself on the following leadership skills and qualities. Use the following scale:
    1 = Strong, need little improvement; 2 = Moderate, need a little work in this area; 3 = Weak, need to focus efforts in this area.

1. _____ I have good interpersonal skills.

2. _____ I am goal oriented.

3. _____ I have a high level of enthusiasm and motivation.

(continues)

(continued)

4. _____ I am able to maintain my focus on the issues.

5. _____ I have a positive outlook and high self-esteem.

6. _____ I can motivate others.

7. _____ I can handle conflict.

8. _____ I tend to focus on solutions as opposed to problems.

Skill Application 8–4 Brainstorming

Using the guidelines from this chapter, set up a small group for brainstorming sessions. Pick a potential opportunity or define a problem about which you would like to generate ideas. Then spend at least 20-minute brainstorming. Try to schedule at least three separate 20-minute sessions.

1. What were the positive outcomes of the brainstorming session? _____

_____

_____

2. What were the negative outcomes of the brainstorming session? _____

_____

_____

3. How would you improve future brainstorming sessions? _____

_____

_____

Cultural Competency and Diversity in the Organization

Cultural competency is defined as the ability to interact effectively with people of different cultures and socioeconomic backgrounds. Cultural competency is vital in the health care setting as it has a positive effect on patient care delivery and outcomes. Health care professionals interact with people of all cultures and backgrounds. It is imperative that respect and compassion be given to all people. Cultural competence is so important that the U.S. Department of Health and Human Services has developed free online continuing education modules for individuals at all levels and in all disciplines of health care.

Skill Application 8–5 Think Cultural Health

Go to https://thinkculturalhealth.hhs.gov/Education/Nurses and choose "Culturally Competent Nursing Care: A Cornerstone of Caring." Register as a new user, and complete the module. Make sure to print the certificate and keep it in a safe place with other certifications you will present to potential employers.

List three things you learned from the module:

_____

_____

_____

Communication and Meetings

Meetings represent another important group interaction that requires good communication skills. Meetings can be held for many reasons. For example, meetings can be used to communicate information, deal with difficult issues, influence attitudes, solve problems, and plan events. Due to the continuing education requirements in health care, often meetings are focused on planning educational programs such as lectures or workshops.

The planning process is critical in ensuring a productive meeting where people feel their attendance was worth their time and effort. The planning process should include who should be invited, the purpose and objectives, and the theme or title of the meeting along with development of a proposed agenda. The location and dates of the meeting should be established as early as possible to reserve the facility and publicize the meeting to the attendees.

As a health care practitioner, you may be required to preside over a meeting. What are some of the things you can do to run a good meeting? First, a warm, personable atmosphere should be established. Refreshments and name tags may be appropriate along with a friendly seating arrangement. At the beginning of the meeting, you should provide a sincere greeting, perform audience introductions if appropriate, and clearly describe the purpose of the meeting. Most meetings are run from an agenda, which lists what is to take place during the meeting. Agendas should minimally include the following:

- Date and time of meeting
- Location of meeting
- Discussion topics
- Any guest speaker or program if applicable

However, more formal business meetings may require a more standardized agenda and standardized way of running the meeting.

Parliamentary procedure is a set of rules, such as *Robert's Rules of Order*, that helps to run larger group meetings and maintain order. In parliamentary procedure, most actions require that a motion be made, seconded, discussed, and then voted on. The motion can be amended (changed) informally if agreement exists with those who made and seconded the motion. Lacking this friendly amendment, a motion can still be made to amend the original motion, but this now needs to be seconded and requires discussion. The amendment is voted upon, after which the main motion is considered again and a vote taken. Did you follow this? This may sound confusing, but after attending a meeting run by these rules, it does make more sense. See Table 8–1 for components of a formal meeting agenda.

Regardless of whether the meeting is formal or informal, the presider of the meeting must be attentive to verbal and nonverbal communication cues. In most meetings, far more is expressed nonverbally than verbally, and presiders can make the meeting more meaningful to more people by being alert to these cues. Are people straining so as to hear or see? Is it too warm or too cold? Is there too much outside distraction? Have people been sitting too long? Is a break needed? Are heads nodding in agreement? Does there seem to be a lot of buzzing about a controversial topic? Is the topic boring, or is it time for a change of format or a change of pace? Is the energy level running low? Are people seemingly anxious to get started on the return trip?

After the meeting concludes, written documentation of what occurred during the meeting must be prepared. This is referred to as the minutes of the meeting. Minutes help to create a history resource for future reference and reminder of decisions made and actions that

Table 8–1
Components of a Formal Meeting Agenda

1.	Call to order
2.	Roll call (if needed)
3.	Approval of minutes of previous meeting
4.	Treasurer's report
5.	Report of officers (if needed)
6.	Report of standing committees (if needed)
7.	Reports of special committees (if needed)
8.	Old business (itemized list)
9.	New business (itemized list)
10.	Program (if there is a program or speaker)
11.	Adjournment

need to be taken. In addition, minutes serve to inform those who did not attend and serve to help form the next meeting's agenda. Minutes should include the following:

- Date and time of meeting
- Members present, absent, and excused
- Acceptance of previous minutes with any corrections
- Announcements
- Concise reporting of discussions, decisions, and actions that need to be taken
- Date, time, and location of next meeting
- Time of adjournment
- Signature of person preparing the minutes and/or the chairperson

Your Clinical Practicum

As a health care professions student, you will be required to spend time in the health care environment as part of your education. This time spent learning is very important. You will be expected to behave in a professional manner. This includes showing up on time, responding well to constructive criticism, and strictly adhering to stated policies such as dress codes. However, a very large part of that professional manner includes appropriate communication within all levels of the organization along with your teachers and fellow students. Very often, health care professions students are hired by the agencies in which they complete the practicum hours. It is very important that you behave in an authentic manner that showcases you in the best possible manner. There are a few things you can do to stand out during your clinical rotations:

- A caring attitude
- Integrity
- Authenticity
- Humility
- Good listening
- Persistence
- Willingness to help

The skills covered in this chapter and throughout this book, when put into practice, will help you achieve success.

Just For

FUN 8-1

Horse Training Applied to People

Work on the same principle as people who train horses. You start with low fences, easily achieved goals, and work up. It's important in management never to ask people to try to accomplish goals they can't accept.

—Ian Mac Gregor

What do you think the speaker means by this statement? Do you think there is a difference between a goal you cannot achieve and a goal you cannot accept?

Summary

- The health care system is a large and varied complex system with many types of organizations outside of the traditional hospital setting. Good communication is vital for success.

- Communication in an organization can sometimes be confusing. One of the best ways to begin to understand the organization is to review the organizational chart and learn the directions of communication flow. This will also aid you in understanding the lines of authority and where you fit into the big picture.

- The grapevine is an informal but very powerful part of any organization.

- To function effectively within any organization, you must understand group dynamics. This will help you identify the types of groups, group goals, and your role within the group.

- Many factors (e.g., communication patterns, cohesiveness, group leadership, and groupthink) can affect group functioning.

- Brainstorming is a great way for groups to generate ideas and begin to interact.

- You will become part of an organization or team regardless of your chosen health care profession. Even if you are independent and run your own business, the business represents an organization, and you will need to understand organizational communication. In addition, the team concept in organization has gained increased emphasis in the newly emerging health care environment.

- Understanding the communication within an organization will keep you connected and informed. This understanding will help you become an integral part of the organization and develop skills that will lead to personal success within the organization.

- These skills need to begin with your clinical practicum and become stronger as you continue in the chosen profession.

- It is important to always be aware and appreciative of those from other cultures than your own.

- Treating patients and other coworkers with respect is vital in ensuring quality outcomes.

Case Study   8–1

You are given the charge to put together a planning committee to develop an educational program for your coworkers on diet and its relationship to diabetes. The objective is to better educate the staff, since they are dealing with an increasing number of patients who have poor dietary habits related to diabetes. List four committee members along with their affiliations or area of expertise. In other words, why would they be effective contributing members of this committee? Remember to bring in as many different perspectives as possible.

Committee member 1: _____

Rationale for their appointment:

_____

_____

Committee member 2: _____

Rationale for their appointment:

Committee member 3: _____

Rationale for their appointment:

_____

Committee member 4: _____

Rationale for their appointment:

_____

_____

Develop an introductory planning meeting agenda for your first meeting.

_____

_____

Internet Activity

Using Internet search engines, find additional material on communication within an organization that can help you and your fellow students. Some suggested keywords are communication channels, chain of command, group dynamics, groupthink, brainstorming, and running meetings. Write down something new that you found to share.

_____

_____

_____

_____

Chapter 9

Patient Interaction and Communication

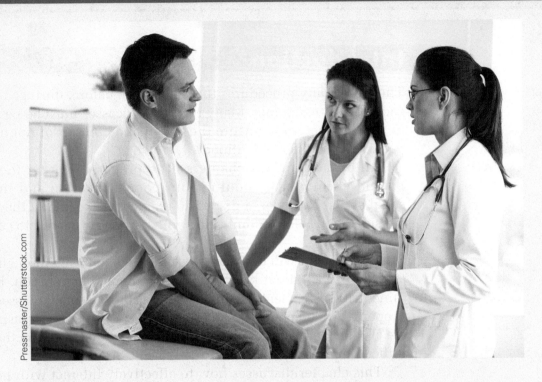

Pressmaster/Shutterstock.com

Objectives

Upon completion of this chapter, you should be able to:

1. Describe ways to properly prepare for the patient encounter.

2. Explain the four stages involved with effective patient interaction.

3. Relate the importance of space and territoriality to the patient encounter.

4. Describe how to satisfy the needs of the patient.

Key Terms

charting

chief complaint or
    chief concern (CC)

documentation

electronic health record (EHR)

Health Insurance Portability and
    Accountability Act (HIPAA)

intimate space

introductory stage

personal space

social space

territoriality

Introduction

A faithful friend is a strong
defense.
A faithful friend is the
medicine of life.

—Apocrypha

There are many procedures that take place before, during, and after each patient encounter. Many thought processes must be performed to near perfection to ensure the safety and comfort of not only the patient but also the practitioner.

All of the previous chapters have prepared you for the initial patient encounter by honing your communication and interpersonal skills. However, a discussion concerning some of the special considerations of communication with patients is needed to complete the picture.

The moment will eventually occur when you walk through a door and there is a patient lying in the room dependent on you. Keep in mind that most patients are not depending on you solely to assess them properly, give them a treatment, or perform other necessary tasks. They are also looking to you as someone to trust and to help them through a difficult time.

This chapter discusses how to effectively interact with patients. Let us begin our journey into one of the most intriguing and rewarding parts of health care—the patient encounter.

Anticipatory Exercise 9–1   Learning the Lingo

Because familiarizing yourself by reading the patient's chart is a first critical step, understanding the medical language of the documentation is crucial. List 10 common medical abbreviations and 10 common medical terms, and define their meanings. Share the results with the class and develop a large master list.

1. Ten medical abbreviations with definitions:

a. _____   f. _____

b. _____   g. _____

c. _____   h. _____

d. _____   i. _____

e. _____   j. _____

(continues)

(continued)

2. Ten medical terms with definitions:

    a. _____   f. _____

    b. _____   g. _____

    c. _____   h. _____

    d. _____   i. _____

    e. _____   j. _____

Preparing for the Patient Encounter

When you successfully graduate from your health care professional program, you will certainly have the academic and clinical skills to place on your resume. However, what will set you apart and what employers are becoming more concerned in assessing is your "soft skills" or "personality skills." Employers realize someone who has good soft skills will communicate and relate well to patients, family members, and fellow health care professionals, and this will only enhance the organizational reputation. This text is about developing and enhancing your soft skills, and this chapter specifically focuses on the importance of good patient interaction skills.

Please note that while this chapter focuses on clinical interactions, it is also important to develop soft skills even if you will not work directly with patients in your health care career. Effective communication is needed for good medical care as it relates to insurance, scheduling, billing, and all areas of customer service.

Before entering a patient's room, several things must be done. One of the first things a health care professional must do is become familiar with the patient. One of the best places to start is the patient's medical record (paper or electronic). The medical record offers you a plethora of information. The medical record is where you will find an almost complete medical history of this person.

You will learn about the patient's reason for seeking medical help. This is often called the patient's **chief complaint or chief concern (CC)**. You will find the patient's name, age, sex, race, and social history (e.g., whether the patient smokes or drinks). You will have a complete medical history and physical to review. Diagnostic tests and treatments are listed with their results. The physician's specific orders are contained in the medical record and must be verified before you perform any specific procedure. Take your time with the medical record, and get to know a lot about the patient. All this information can facilitate the creation of a bond between the professional and the patient.

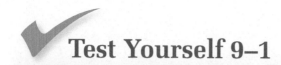

Test Yourself 9–1

Medical Lingo

Medical records contain many medical abbreviations and terminology that represent a unique language. You must be able to understand this language to effectively understand the medical record and communicate with others. See how many of the following common terms you know.

STAT _____   OOB _____

MOM _____   NKA _____

BID _____   NPO _____

PRN _____   CPR _____

SOB _____   TID _____

Answers can be found in Appendix F.

Other things that are important to know and understand are any special precautions that need to be taken. For example, is the patient NPO (nothing by mouth) due to surgery? This would be very important to know if the patient asked you for a glass of juice. Is the patient allowed out of bed? Must the patient remain flat because of spinal surgery? Should you take any special precautions to prevent the spread of the disease? As stated previously, get to know your patient not only so that you can communicate more effectively with them but also so that you can alleviate risks and potentially life-threatening situations.

At this time, you can also talk to other health care professionals who have interacted with this patient (Figure 9–1). They may be able

Figure 9–1
Review the patient record and confer with other professionals concerning your patient.

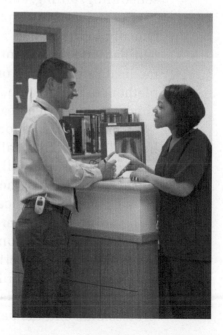

to give you an idea of the patient's mental state and compliance with treatments. A recent progress note on the chart will also indicate the patient's current status.

The Actual Patient Encounter

Now that you have learned everything you need to know about your patient, it is time for the initial patient encounter. Sometimes, you are never really prepared for what you are going to find when entering the room, but you handle things as they are brought to you in a professional manner. For example, is your patient going to be in a good mood or bad mood? Is your patient going to be awake or unconscious? Just take things in stride, and do your job well.

Just For

FUN 9–1

Reflections

Courage, love, friendship, compassion, and empathy lift us above the simple beasts and define humanity.

—The Book of Counted Sorrows

Write in your own words what you think this quotation means and how it may pertain to the health professional and their encounters with patients. Be prepared to discuss it in class.

At first, you may feel overwhelmed with communicating with your patient while also performing a proper assessment and treatment. This may all seem like too much to remember at once. What do you do first? Take heart in the fact that eventually everything will flow together, and you will develop a smooth routine with practice over time.

To help you understand the "flow" of events that occur, the patient encounter can be broken down into the following four stages:

1. The introductory stage
2. Patient assessment
3. Treating and monitoring the patient
4. Feedback and follow-up

Stage 1: The Introductory Stage

The **introductory stage** may be considered one of the most vital stages in setting the initial tone of how your patient will perceive you. When you enter the room, the patient may already be wary of you and your intentions. The patient may have been in the hospital for some time now and may be tired of being poked and prodded by different people. This is one reason why it was necessary to research your patient, because it is now time to develop a rapport with your patient.

When you enter the room, formally introduce yourself to your patient and explain who you are and why you are there. For example: "Hello, Mr. Saloom, my name is Tina, and I'm a respiratory therapist. I'm here to give you your breathing treatment this morning." In time, the patient will get to know you and may allow you to use their first name. Sometimes you will have patients who are comatose, and you may not see the need for addressing them, but there is a need. These patients are still human and should also be addressed and given any explanation on care and treatments.

The introductory stage is when the patient makes their first impression of you. Therefore, it is a good idea to get off to a positive start. If you present yourself in a negative manner or with a false pretense, the patient will sense this. In this situation, the patient may lack trust in your ability to provide treatment. If this happens, things may not go too smoothly the entire time you have this individual as a patient.

You should enter the room in a positive frame of mind. Be friendly but not overly friendly because this may be interpreted as fake. Be professional in the way you act and speak. If a patient asks you a question, answer it to the best of your ability. Another important aspect of patient interaction is eye contact. Do not look out the window when the patient speaks. Look directly at the patient and show that person that you are interested and concerned about their thoughts and feelings. Also watch what you say in certain situations. Some patients may be in the hospital for an extended period and may be depressed about their circumstances. You may not help the patient's state of mind if you enter the room and say, "Oh, Mr. Little, it is so beautiful out. The sun is shining, and I can't wait to go golfing." How do you think Mr. Little may feel?

All in all, if you present yourself positively, things will go well; but then again, you will have patients who are difficult to deal with no matter how you present yourself. They may be uninterested in what you have to say or do, and sometimes they may be resistive. Once again, be yourself in these situations and do your job to the utmost. Sometimes you may have to try a little harder with these patients, and they may come around to you.

The number one thing is to show that you care and that you are there because you want to be, not because you have to be. These patients especially need a friendly and professional caregiver to help them through this difficult time in their life.

Food for Thought 9–1

How Would You React?

Often you will develop close relationships with your patients. They may even confide in you with very personal and private information. How would you handle the following situation?

A female pediatric patient has been very withdrawn. However, she has grown close to you and looks forward to her treatment and her interaction with you. You even help her give a treatment to her teddy bear. One day she tells you that she is being sexually abused at home. How would you handle this? What if you got nervous and quickly left the room and avoided the issue? Do you think she would ever develop the courage to tell anyone else?

Stage 2: Patient Assessment

During patient assessment, you will evaluate the condition of your patient. You will look at the patient's overall appearance, reaction toward you, personality, and attitude. With practice and as your comfort level increases, you will learn how to assess your patient the first moment you walk in the room and begin speaking.

When you assess the patient, you are looking for information that indicates the current health status. This includes inspection of the patient's general appearance and color. Is the patient cyanotic (blue) or jaundiced (yellow-orange)? Is the patient having labored respirations? Does the patient appear confused or anxious? With practice and knowledge, you will soon rival Sherlock Holmes with your inspection skills.

Besides inspection, you may also assess the patient's vital signs, palpate and percuss certain areas, and auscultate the lungs. All the while, you are noting any changes in the patient's physical appearance and watching for any signs of difficulty the patient may be having due to their condition. This initial assessment will give you a baseline of data to compare after the treatment. Having this information will help you note changes in the patient's condition. A proper assessment will also aid you in determining whether the treatment prescribed for the patient is appropriate and effective in treating this patient's condition.

Stage 3: Treating and Monitoring the Patient

You have checked the physician's orders for the prescribed treatment and reviewed the chart. You have introduced yourself, assessed the patient, and determined that the treatment is appropriate and necessary. You also now have a data baseline for this patient before intervening with treatment. Now it is time to actually begin the treatment. While you are administering the treatment, you will need to monitor and assess your patient. Monitoring the patient's vital signs and reactions throughout the procedure is critical for the patient's safety. If you see any discrepancies from the initial vitals or if the patient seems to be in any distress, stop the procedure immediately and contact the attending nurse and the patient's physician to communicate the situation.

During the treatment stage, you need to give positive reinforcement and encouragement to your patient. Praise the patient for doing a good job and give assurance that all is going well. Encourage the patient to give their best effort during a treatment that requires patient participation. Remember to explain in lay terms why the treatment is being administered and what it will accomplish.

Stage 4: Feedback and Follow-Up

Once you have performed all the necessary tasks, it is time to assess the patient one more time to see how the patient is post-treatment. Check the vital signs again, and most important, ask the patient how they are feeling. Does the patient feel better, the same, or worse? You are going to want to note all these items on the patient's chart for future reference.

Give your patient specific feedback about how well they did with the treatment. Make any appropriate suggestions that would improve the effectiveness of the treatment. Leave with a pleasant, courteous farewell such as, "Thank you, Mrs. Jones, I hope you have a nice afternoon." If you are scheduled to return, let your patient know that you will be back to see them.

Now that the patient encounter is over, it is time to record all the procedures that were performed. You will want to document how the treatment went, how the patient responded to the treatment, the vital signs, the treatment or procedures performed on the patient, and so on. The following is an example of how a respiratory treatment may be documented:

> *Aerosol treatment × 10 minutes with 0.5 cc albuterol and CPT to left upper lobe × 7 minutes. Breath sounds pre- and post-treatment—rhonchi bilaterally. HR 78–80–79. Patient had productive cough with moderate amount of thick, yellow mucus. Patient tolerated treatment well. Returned to 3 liter O$_2$ via nasal cannula.*
>
> *G. Perry, RRT*

Charting or **documentation** is essential to health care. If a malpractice case were to be filed, the health record could be your best friend. It will show the date and time you performed the procedure, and all the therapies performed. This is why it is good to include as much detail as possible and also to assess your patient's status to the fullest.

Each patient has a health record, which is a legal record that contains biographical data, medical histories, physician orders, physical exam and diagnostic test results, and assessment and progress notes from various health care disciplines. Due to the personal and sometimes sensitive information contained in a health record or during conversations between health care professionals, confidentiality must be maintained. All information given to a health care professional or contained in a health record is considered privileged communication and by law must only be shared with other members of the patient's health care team unless a written consent of permission is given by the patient. There are certain exceptions to this law such as the requirement to report communicable or sexually transmitted diseases and injuries caused by violence that require law enforcement involvement. This law is the **Health Insurance Portability and Accountability Act (HIPAA)**.

Here are some important aspects to documenting:

- Always document the date and time; in the **electronic health record (EHR)**, there will be an automatic time stamp applied.
- Deleting information in charts is not allowed; corrections can be made in accordance with your facility policy.
- Charting should be in concise, objective, and accurate language. (Do not interject personal feelings or derogatory statements.)
- Abbreviations are allowed if on your organization's approved list.
- Only document what you have done; do not chart for someone else.
- Check for the right patient, the right health record, and that you are using the right form.

Note that most health care facilities use military or international time, not the traditional time used in everyday life. Military time avoids the confusion between A.M. and P.M. used in traditional time. For example, if just 4:30 had been written and the A.M. or P.M. was omitted, you would not know if this was 4:30 in the morning or afternoon. Military time uses 0100 (1:00 A.M. traditional time) through 2400 (12:00 A.M. midnight traditional time). For example, 1630 would represent 4:30 P.M. Please see Table 9–1, which shows the conversion between military and traditional time.

Computerized Documentation. With the common use of computers and computerized charting, additional safeguards must be implemented to prevent others from viewing confidential information. Computer access should be limited to only those health care professionals who should be viewing this information. Using codes and requiring passwords are additional ways to safeguard against unwanted access. Attending orientation training and sessions for any updates to the system will make this process go smoothly. While computerized charting systems do vary, keep in mind to double-check to make sure that you have entered the correct patient identification code, and document or access information only in your authorized areas. Finally, do not share your password with anyone else.

Table 9–1
Military (24-Hour Clock) and Traditional Time Conversion Chart

Traditional Time Morning	Military Time	Traditional Time Afternoon	Military Time
12:01 A.M.	0001	12:01 P.M.	1201
12:30 A.M.	0030	12:30 P.M.	1230
1:00 A.M.	0100	1:00 P.M.	1300
2:00 A.M.	0200	2:00 P.M.	1400
3:00 A.M.	0300	3:00 P.M.	1500
4:00 A.M.	0400	4:00 P.M.	1600
5:00 A.M.	0500	5:00 P.M.	1700
6:00 A.M.	0600	6:00 P.M.	1800
7:00 A.M.	0700	7:00 P.M.	1900
8:00 A.M.	0800	8:00 P.M.	2000
9:00 A.M.	0900	9:00 P.M.	2100
10:00 A.M.	1000	10:00 P.M.	2200
11:00 A.M.	1100	11:00 P.M.	2300
12:00 noon	1200	12:00 midnight	2400

Food for Thought 9–2

The Patient's World

The patient's *world* becomes the hospital room, especially if they have been in the hospital for an extended period. The patient may not be allowed out of bed, and therefore, the items on the nightstand (e.g., glasses, tissues) are very important and need to be within reach. Therefore, before leaving the patient's room, put anything you may have moved during the encounter back to where it was.

How do you think a nonambulatory patient would feel if you moved the nightstand before doing the treatment and then forget to return it to within reach? What will this do to your rapport with this patient? What are some other ways that you can respect the patient's world (room)?

Skill Application 9–1 Mock Patient Encounters

Work with a partner and pretend that one of you is the patient and one the health care professional. Develop a script that has the health care professional go through all the components of the patient encounter, including the introduction, history taking, assessment, vital signs, and a mock treatment. Each group will then perform its skit for the class, and the class will critique the encounter. Each group should have at least one thing done wrong (e.g., forgetting to put the nightstand back) or some unusual characteristic (e.g., a noncompliant patient). See if the class can identify the wrong or unusual circumstance.

Skill Application 9–2 **The SOAPIE Note**

There is a specific type of nursing progress note called the SOAPIE note. Using your research skills, investigate what a SOAPIE note is and give an example of an actual note.

1. What is a SOAPIE note? _____

2. Give an example of a SOAPIE note. _____

   S: _____

   O: _____

   A: _____

   P: _____

   I: _____

   E: _____

Respecting a Patient's Space

Space is a very important aspect of communication that is often overlooked or disregarded in the patient encounter. A patient's room usually becomes a temporary home, and it is necessary for you to respect that patient's territory and individual space. There are three basic categories of space:

- **Social space**
- **Personal space**
- **Intimate space**

Understanding the boundaries and special characteristics of these spaces will enhance your ability to communicate with your patient.

Social Space

Social space is defined as the distance of 4 to 12 feet from the patient. This is where it is most appropriate for you to introduce yourself to the patient and begin the communication process (Figure 9–2). You will be able to see the entire room and patient at this distance and develop a sense of awareness for where everything belongs.

As stated, this is the space for the introductions, but limit what you say because others are in range to hear what you say. Giving confidential or personal information within this space would violate the patient's trust in your confidentiality. Your approach should be more formal in nature at this point.

Figure 9–2
Social space is 4 to
12 feet from the patient.

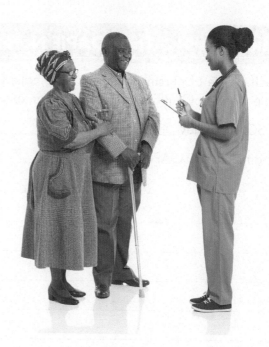

Personal Space

Personal space is defined as approximately 18 inches to 4 feet between you and the patient. After introducing yourself in the social space, you will move to the personal space, usually at the patient's side (Figure 9–3). You are now close enough to the patient at this time to conduct a personal interview without anyone overhearing and at the same time far enough away from the patient so as not to make them feel uncomfortable or awkward.

This is the space where you tell the patient about the treatment or ask specific questions concerning the condition. Not only will your body position, manner of speaking, and facial expressions add to the impression, but your general appearance will also. Patients will have more faith in a person who is clean and presentable than in a person who is unkempt and dirty.

Figure 9–3
Personal space is
18 inches to 4 feet away
from the patient.

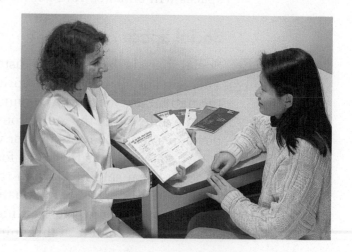

This is the space in which you are developing trust with the patient. As stated previously, it is important that communication between you and your patient go smoothly so as to develop trust. Once trust is established, it is easier for you to approach and invade the patient's intimate space, where your assessment and treatment will take place.

Intimate Space

Intimate space is the area about 0 to 18 inches away from the patient. Whereas personal space still allowed patient comfort, invasion of the intimate space can sometimes be awkward for the patient. It is helpful to explain to the patient what you are going to do and why before proceeding with activities in the intimate space. This may improve the patient's comfort level (Figure 9–4).

Intimate space is where you will perform the physical examination of the patient. During this period, there is little eye contact and communication between the patient and the practitioner. Only instruction to the patient is needed during this intimate encounter and performance of the assessment. The instructions should be short and to the point.

The time spent in the patient's intimate space should be relatively short. Perform the physical examination as quickly and thoroughly as possible. Many factors, such as the patient's health status, age, and gender, may play a limiting role in the tasks you can perform. You may want to work more slowly and carefully with certain patients.

Respecting the patient's space by beginning in the social and personal spaces and then performing assessments and treatments that invade the intimate space will establish trust with your patient. Can you imagine how you would feel if someone walked into your hospital room and immediately began to take your vital signs or auscultate your lungs without any introductions?

Figure 9–4
Intimate space is 0 to 18 inches away from the patient.

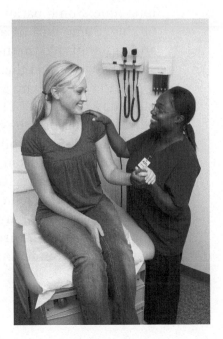

Territoriality

Territoriality is a major factor in relationships with others. People claim certain space or territory as their own. The patient's room over time becomes their turf, or territory. When you enter the patient's room, take notice of where the patient has everything placed. As stated previously, during the treatment, you may have to move things to facilitate the tasks you are performing. Once you finish these tasks, make sure you put everything back where it was. If you move a chair, put it back. Sometimes you may forget, but most likely the next time you see that patient, they will say something to you about it.

Putting items back may not be a big deal to you, but it is to the patient. This is the patient's room, and for a lot of patients, it has become home. Patients need to be able to reach things such as their glasses or hearing aids because some may be confined to bed. Keep all of these things in mind during patient encounters. Sooner rather than later, it will all become second nature.

Territoriality is also important at the nurses' station or medical office. If you remove a chart from a specific area, put it back. For example, charts may be placed in a certain area after a physician writes orders. If you remove a chart from this area for your review and return it to the chart rack, you may seriously delay the implementation of critical procedures or medications.

Patient Needs

Many patients you will encounter may have been hospitalized for a long time. Some patients will be comatose; others will be alert and talking. Some will be as pleasant as can be; others will be grumpy and agitated. No matter what type of patient you encounter, you should always treat that person in a professional manner.

In 1943, Abraham Maslow developed a theory called "Maslow's hierarchy of needs." This theory states that people need their basic needs met before they can move on to meet higher level needs (see Figure 9–5). Hospitalized patients are often in need of the basic physiological needs: air, food, and water. This is important to keep in mind when dealing with patients who are sick or injured.

Being hospitalized can be one of the most traumatic experiences of a person's life. Many patients become depressed and lose faith. Their life has been turned upside down. They cannot function as they usually would. Sometimes they wake in the morning exhausted

Figure 9–5
Hospitalized patients are often seeking to fulfill their physiological needs.

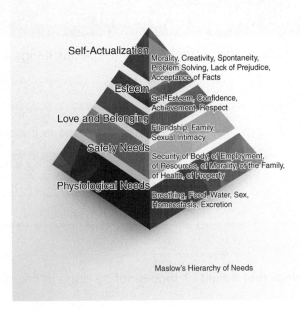

Self-Actualization — Morality, Creativity, Spontaneity, Problem Solving, Lack of Prejudice, Acceptance of Facts

Esteem — Self-Esteem, Confidence, Achievement, Respect

Love and Belonging — Friendship, Family, Sexual Intimacy

Safety Needs — Security of Body, of Employment, of Resources, of Morality, of the Family, of Health, of Property

Physiological Needs — Breathing, Food, Water, Sex, Homeostasis, Excretion

Maslow's Hierarchy of Needs

because of being awakened at night for medication and treatments. They look forward to having visitors, but sometimes their families and friends cannot make it that day. Some of the patients may have no family at all. These are all factors you must consider. Sometimes you have to think how you would feel if you were that patient. Loneliness and depression can affect the progress of the patient. This is where a health care professional can play a major role in a patient's recovery. Even if the patient's circumstance is terminal, the health care professional can still try to bring a smile to the patient's face. Talk to your patients, check on them throughout the day, and ask how they are feeling and if they need anything. You have already established a rapport; now give them a pillar to lean on, someone to talk to, and someone to listen. You will develop many meaningful relationships with your patients that will add to not only their lives but also your own.

One final but very important reminder is that health care professionals will encounter various cultural differences in their patient population. It is important to learn about the cultures that exist within your geographical region because this will help you to deliver high-quality care. Chapter 8 asked you to complete an online cultural competency module; if you have not yet completed this, please do so now. This will also help you to enrich and improve your own life by appreciating that there are many valid approaches to what someone believes, not only in health care and healing but also in their views on life.

Skill Application 9–3 Types of Space

List the three types of space, and give three specific things that should or should not be done within each space.

1. Type of space: _____

    Three things that should or should not be done in this space:

    a. _____

    b. _____

    c. _____

2. Type of space: _____

    Three things that should or should not be done in this space:

    a. _____

    b. _____

    c. _____

3. Type of space: _____

    Three things that should or should not be done in this space:

    a. _____

    b. _____

    c. _____

Skill Application 9–4 Assessing Meeting Patient Needs

Select two skills from Table 9–2 found on the following page that you feel you can improve upon and develop an action plan to accomplish.

Skill #1 _____

Action Plan

_____

_____

_____

_____

(continues)

(continued)

Skill #2 _____

Action Plan

_____

_____

_____

_____

Please see Table 9–2, which gives a brief summary of the top skills needed for good patient interaction and communication. These skills will help you fully meet the needs of the patients within your care.

Table 9–2
Top Skills Needed for Effective Patient Interaction and Meeting Patient Needs

Skill	Description
Empathy	Understanding the patient's perspective and expressing that understanding through respect and support in the form of feelings, concern, or ideas is empathy.
Positive attitude	A positive attitude is maintaining a cheerful and welcoming attitude. This attitude can become "contagious" and carry over to your patients, their families, and fellow workers.
Good work ethic	A good work ethic shows you have a value set based on hard work, professionalism, punctuality, teamwork, and motivation to do your best. This is needed in the health care professions, which can be very demanding with sometimes long hours.
Flexibility	Flexibility is the ability to adapt. It is needed for handling the ever-changing health care environment, which will most likely offer something different each day. You will also need to be flexible in your work schedule as you might be on call or have to stay later on your shift due to an emergency.
Stress management	Health care is a demanding career and your ability to handle stress will save you from burnout. Burnout is long-term exhaustion and loss of interest in your work. Stress management is so important that Chapter 5 is dedicated to it.
Time management	Time management is organizing your work in an efficient manner and setting appropriate priorities. This is needed when you are sometimes pulled in different directions by various demands or have to prioritize treatment such as in triage.
Confidence	Projecting confidence in your skills will directly communicate and influence the patient's experience in a positive manner.
Receptive attitude	A receptive attitude means you can handle constructive criticism in a positive manner and make corrective changes when needed. Health care knowledge and advances seem to double every few years, so it is important to have a receptive attitude to learning new information and techniques.

Summary

- Patient interaction may be the most difficult yet rewarding part of your health care profession.

- It is important to prepare for your inter-action with the patient by assessing the patient's health record and getting all the background information and facts that will facilitate your interaction.

- The next step is called the introductory stage; during this stage, you introduce yourself and establish a positive impression in the patient's mind.

- The assessment stage follows, during which you evaluate the patient's condition using the assessment skills that you have mastered.

- The third stage is the treatment and monitoring stage. It is important to give reinforcement and encouragement during this stage.

- The final stage is the feedback and follow-up stage, when the patient is told how they are doing with the treatment and the results are recorded in the patient's chart.

- Space is an important consideration in treating patients. The three types of space include social, personal, and intimate space.

- Social space (4 to 12 feet between you and the patient) is for preliminary introductions.

- Personal space (18 inches to 4 feet between you and the patient) is reserved for the personal interview and discussions.

- Intimate space (0 to 18 inches between you and the patient) is where you will perform the physical examination and many thera-peutic treatments.

- Whatever health care profession you choose, you will learn how to perform all the therapeutic techniques and diagnostic tests associated with your profession. This knowledge and the particular areas of emphasis vary among professions. How-ever, what does not vary is the interaction with patients. Establishing an effective rapport with your patient can greatly influence compliance with treatments and even the outcome of the disease or problem.

- It is critical that you apply all the communication skills that you have learned and practiced thus far to the actual patient encounter. This advance prepara-tion and understanding will help your first encounter go much more smoothly than if you had not prepared. However, it may take a while and several patients before you feel totally comfortable with your interaction. This is natural, and we all go through it.

Case Study 9–1

You are assigned to do quality control for your department. Part of this responsibility is reviewing health records to make sure that proper documentation procedures are being followed by staff members. Review the following entry and see if you can identify four mistakes with this charting entry.

Date: 6-24-24 Time 4:30

Patient was given instructions on proper wound care by Mary Beth for 30 to 60 minutes. Patient wasn't very bright and it took longer than normal to teach the proper procedure.

Charted by Rich Jones

Mistake #1 _____

Mistake #2 _____

Mistake #3 _____

Mistake #4 _____

Answers can be found in Appendix F.

Internet Activity

Using Internet search engines, find additional material on patient interaction and communication that can help you and your fellow students. Some suggested keywords are interviewing patients, medical charting, computerized charting, territoriality, and types of social space. Write down something new that you found to share.

_____

_____

_____

_____

Chapter 10

Your First Position as a Health Care Professional

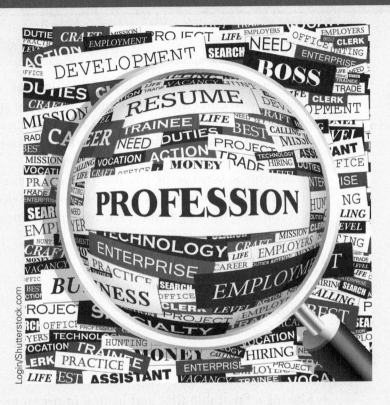

Login/Shutterstock.com

Objectives

Upon completion of this chapter, you should be able to:

1. Perform the steps needed to secure a rewarding career.

2. Develop an effective résumé.

3. Locate the available positions that fit your skills.

4. Develop a cover letter.

5. Prepare for the interview process.

6. Define the skills needed to succeed in the interview process.

7. Define the characteristics, attitudes, and interpersonal skills needed to succeed in the workplace.

8. Relate the importance of professional image to career success.

Key Terms

behavioral interview	empathy	punctuality
competency	functional résumé	respect
cover letter	interview	résumé
emotional intelligence (EI)	professional image	trust

Introduction

Learning isn't a means to an end; it is an end itself.

—Robert A. Heinlein

You have worked hard in school and showcased yourself in order to become a health care professional. You have spent hours learning theories, practicing techniques in the lab, doing research, and working with patients. Your hard work will now pay off in the form of your first job as a health care professional.

There are several steps you need to take after graduation to ensure that your first position will be the start of a challenging and personally rewarding lifelong career. These steps include the following:

- Choosing the type of position you wish to secure
- Preparing your résumé
- Making contacts and finding openings
- Writing a cover letter
- Applying to positions
- Interviewing
- Accepting a position
- Making a favorable first and lasting impression

This chapter takes an in-depth look at each of these steps. Remember, the time and effort you spend on each of these steps will influence the final outcome of the position you receive. Figure 10–1 shows the steps to a rewarding career.

Choosing the Right Position

There are numerous areas of employment and types of positions for a health care professional. For example, you can work in the traditional hospital setting or a rehabilitation unit, or you can perform home care. Opportunities exist in physician offices, outpatient clinics, and surgical units. Skilled nursing facilities and the armed forces offer additional opportunities as do medical and pharmaceutical sales positions. You should choose an initial position that suits your talents and interests. Some students are obtaining a degree that places them directly into a role (e.g., medical laboratory technician) while others are getting a more broad degree that will allow them to look at many different types of positions. See Table 10–1 for a listing of possible job opportunities in health care. Can you think of any to add to the list?

Figure 10–1
The steps to a rewarding career.

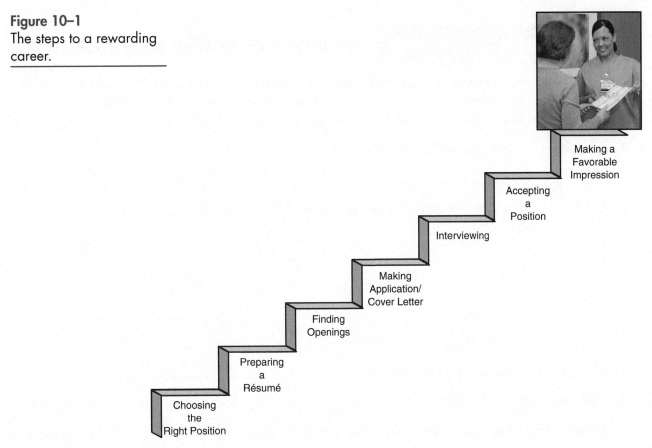

Making a Favorable Impression

Accepting a Position

Interviewing

Making Application/ Cover Letter

Finding Openings

Preparing a Résumé

Choosing the Right Position

Table 10–1
Careers in Healthcare

Anesthesiologist assistant/technician	Massage therapists
Athletic trainer	Medical assistant
Audiologist	Medical transcriptionist
Cardiovascular technician	Nursing (registered nurse [RN], licensed practical nurse [LPN], nursing assistant [NA], patient care technician [PCT])
Behavioral health assistant/technician	Nuclear medicine technologist
Clinical laboratory staff	Occupational or physical therapy assistant
Cytotechnology	Ophthalmic assistants/technicians
Radiology technician (MRI, CT scan, mammography, ultrasound, etc.)	Orthotics and prosthetics assistants/technicians
Dental hygiene/assistant/laboratory technician	Perfusionist
Sonography	Pharmacy technicians/assistants
Food service (dietitians, technicians, assistants, nutritionists)	Podiatry assistants
Emergency medical technician	Polysomnographic technologist
Exercise science	Recreation therapy assistants
Health information technology (medical coders, medical records technicians)	Rehabilitation service workers
Histotechnologist	Respiratory therapy
Home health (HHAs, PCAs, LPNs, RNs)	Blood bank specialist/technicians
Medical insurance billing specialist	Surgical technologist

Anticipatory Exercise 10–1   What Type of Position Suits You?

The answers to the following questions will help you target the type of initial health care position that maximizes your chance for success. These interests may change over time and periodically need to be reassessed. For now, how would you answer the following?

1. Is there a particular region or climate in which you wish to live?

   _____

2. In what type of organization would you like to work (large, small, or do you want to be self-employed)?

   _____

3. Do you like working with any particular type of patient (specific disease or age)?

   _____

4. What type of salary range is acceptable to you? _____

5. What benefits are essential to you? _____

6. How important is job security? _____

7. What is it about your profession that really excites you? _____

Taking a careful inventory of your skills, interests, and experience can help you hone in on the right position for you. For example, you may love to work with infants and children. A children's hospital or a neonatal unit may be a place that interests you.

Skill Application 10–1 What Type of Position Do You Desire?

Before looking in earnest for your job, take some time and get a visual picture of just what type of job you desire. Look at your answers to the "Anticipatory Exercise" questions in the chapter. Now list the top five attributes of your ideal position. Keep these in mind as you search.

a. _____

b. _____

c. _____

d. _____

e. _____

Preparing a Résumé

Now that you have an idea of what type of position you want, you are ready to start job hunting. Sometimes in health care, you are fortunate enough to have a position before you graduate. However, this is not always the case, and you can expect to look for weeks or months before finding that ideal position. Do not become discouraged; if you are properly prepared, you will find successful employment. To become properly prepared, a résumé is needed.

A **résumé** is a short summary that highlights "who you are." It tells a potential employer about your education, experience, and qualifications for the job. The résumé is often the first screening tool used by an employer to determine whether the applicant warrants an interview. Therefore, it is essential that your résumé be accurate, complete, neat, and error free. This shows that you took pride in preparing this résumé and are likely to take pride in your work as a potential employee.

Organizing your résumé so that information is easily obtained is important. At this point in your career, the information should be kept to one page but not so crowded that it all runs together. Use of white space is important to separate headings.

The information on a résumé is listed in reverse chronological order. For example, the most recent job or degree held is listed first, followed by other jobs or degrees in reverse chronological order. As a new graduate, you may have little work experience. Therefore, you can develop more of a **functional résumé**. A functional résumé lists your experience in terms of skills you have used on the job or throughout your educational career. To save space, write your information in phrases rather than complete sentences. Get help in preparing your résumé. Ask a knowledgeable person to edit and proofread it; checking with your college career resource center is a great place to start. Make sure to save your résumé as a word document so that you can edit it as needed. It may be tempting to use an online template to create your resume. These are often not readable by the electronic systems used by employers to screen resumes. You should use Microsoft Word to create your resume.

Your résumé should minimally include the following:

- Your name, permanent address, e-mail address, and telephone number.
- Your employment objective; this should be one line and adjusted to match job openings.
- Your education, including school names and addresses, dates you attended, type of program, degree(s) or certificate(s) received, and any honors; you only need to add your grade point average if it is above 3.0.
- Your work experience—paid or volunteer. (For each job, include job title, name and address of employer, and dates of employment. Your skills can be listed here or in another separate section.)

- Any professional licenses and their expiration dates.
- Military experience, including branch and length of service, major responsibilities, and special training.
- Membership in organizations.
- Special skills, foreign languages, honors, awards, and achievements.

An outdated practice is to state "References Available upon Request" at the conclusion of your résumé. This statement is not necessary; however, make sure that you have at least three references with contact information (including phone and e-mail) listed on a separate sheet of paper in case they are requested or needed to fill out the job application. You must always ask permission of the person you wish to use as a reference. Some employers ask you to fill in an electronic form or upload your resume and have it populate the fields. Always double-check that the information being pulled from your resume is where you want it on the electronic form before hitting submit.

Skill Application 10–2 Developing Your Résumé

Your résumé is certainly an item that should be included in your portfolio. Remember, your résumé represents you "on paper" to your potential employer. Using what you have learned in this text, coupled with any outside help you can find, complete your résumé. Develop your résumé and save so that you can periodically update it. Use the following checklist as a review, and check each completed item.

My résumé is:

_____ Neat

_____ Accurate

_____ Well organized

_____ Error free

_____ Comprehensive, containing all the information listed in this chapter

Making Contacts and Finding Openings

Having prepared a résumé, you are now ready to find job openings that match your employment objective. You can receive information concerning potential jobs from a variety of sources. Some examples of formal sources include the following:

- Professional journals and magazine ads
- School placement services
- The Internet (LinkedIn, company websites, or job sites like Indeed.com)
- Job fairs

Figure 10–2 shows a sample functional résumé.

KELLY CISNEROS
9125 Soledad Avenue
El Paso, TX 79907
(915) 123-4567
kcisneros@gmail.com

OBJECTIVE | Position as a **Medical Assistant** in a pediatric office

EDUCATION
AS Degree, Medical Assistant, 2022
Caldwell Technical College, El Paso
• Perfect Attendance Award three semesters out of four
• Grade point average 3.8/4.0
• Externship at Valley Pediatric Center, El Paso
• "Excellent Rating" for overall externship performance

EXPERIENCE WITH CHILDREN
6 years providing private daycare in home
3 years teaching disabled preschoolers
Cub Scout leader
Volunteer tutor at Sanchez Elementary School

ORGANIZATIONAL SKILLS
Maintained state-approved daycare facility
Secretary of PTA at children's school
Coordinate scheduling and activities for local junior soccer team

COMMUNICATION SKILLS
Make presentations to local organizations about child safety issues
Write articles for Sanchez Elementary School parent newsletter
5 years experience as telephone receptionist in a busy insurance office
Speak, read, and write Spanish fluently

WORK HISTORY
Cisneros Quality Daycare 2014–2020
Owner of home-based daycare for up to six children

SpecialCare Preschool   2011–2014
Teacher

Calderon Insurance Agency   2006–2011
Receptionist

Figure 10–2
A sample functional résumé.

You can also search by contacting people you know within the health care profession. Many times, they can provide you with inside leads. This informal type of networking is very effective, especially when you extend it to people that your parents, relatives, friends, and fellow students know.

If you have a particular place you desire to work but the organization has no published openings, you should still make contact. Direct contact with a potential employer can provide the organization with a positive impression of your desire and enthusiasm for working there. This will keep you in the employer's mind and give you a possible advantage when the next opening appears. Remember, the more active you are in searching, the more potential opportunities you will identify.

Skill Application 10–3 Making Contacts

List at least five contacts that can help you find a potential job. These can include individuals or Internet sites.

a. _____

b. _____

c. _____

d. _____

e. _____

Writing Cover Letters

Now that you have a quality résumé in hand and have identified several potential employers, your next step is to prepare a **cover letter**. The cover letter demonstrates your interest in a particular job and working for a particular employer. Unlike your résumé, which can be copied and sent out to several employers, your cover letter must be specific and unique for each job. Its purpose is to get the employer to review your résumé and call you in for an interview. The cover letter should imply that this is "the position" you really want. Major points concerning the cover letter include the following:

- The cover letter should be one page.

- Address the letter to a specific person. Call and find out who that person is versus sending it "To Whom It May Concern." Make sure that you spell the person's name correctly!

- State the purpose of the letter in the first paragraph.
- Elaborate on why your skills and experience match the job.
- Show why you are the person for the position and the value you can add to the organization.
- In summation, ask for an interview and state where and when you can be reached.
- Make the cover letter neat, well organized, error free, and positive.

The cover letter and résumé will get you to the next step in the process—the interview. You may also be requested to fill out an employer application before the interview. Therefore, it is a good idea to bring along a copy of your résumé to serve as a resource when filling out the application. This will demonstrate your preparedness and responsibility. Figure 10–3 shows a sample cover letter.

Skill Application 10–4 The Cover Letter

Again, using what you have learned from your text and outside sources, and figure 10–3 on the following page as a guide develop a cover letter to one of the contacts mentioned in the previous activity (10–3).

The Interview

You have now impressed a future potential employee "on paper." The next step is to see how you interact personally and professionally. The **interview** allows the employer to evaluate your career potential skills, knowledge, character, and oral communication skills. In essence, the employer is trying to determine whether you are the best employee for the position. The interview is your chance to make a good first impression not only to land the position but also to set the tone for how well you will be received on the job. Therefore, it is critical that you take the time to properly prepare for the interview process.

The interview can be separated into three stages. The *preinterview* stage is when you learn all you can about your potential job and employer. This is the time to research the organizational goals, vision, and mission statement. You learn about your department and how it fits into the "big picture." You also learn about your position and what is expected of you. You can search the company website to

Position Advertisement

DENTAL ASSISTANT. Excellent verbal, scheduling and collection skills. Full-time. Front and back office as needed. Computer literate with good work ethic. Commitment to high-quality patient care.

1357 Keystone Drive
Chicago, IL 60606
July 23, 2024

Dr. Harold Mims
1842 Grand Avenue
Chicago, IL 60606

Dear Dr. Mims:

This letter is in response to your advertisement for a dental assistant. I recently graduated from Harrison Dental College and believe that I fulfill the requirements stated in your ad.

Providing **high-quality patient** care was emphasized throughout the dental assisting program at Harrison. I would welcome the opportunity to begin my dental assisting career in an environment where patients are the top priority.

The program at Harrison emphasized the need for good **verbal skills** in the workplace. We were given many opportunities to practice them. In the skills lab students were required to explain all procedures orally to "patients" before and during hands-on work. I also received grades of "A" in my communication courses, which included Oral Communication and Interpersonal Relations for the Health Care Worker.

I understand the need for a smooth-running **front office** and enjoyed the administrative and **computer training** portion of my training. Performing duties in both the **front and back office** would allow me to apply my organizational skills. My previous jobs, outlined in the enclosed résumé, required me to be responsive to the needs of my employers.

My **strong work ethic** is demonstrated in my excellent attendance records, both at school and work, willingness to complete all assigned tasks, and commitment to doing my best at all times.

I would appreciate the opportunity to meet with you to further discuss how I might contribute to the success of your practice. I can be reached at (312) 123-4567.

Thank you for your consideration.

Sincerely,

Kelly Bosner

Kelly Bosner

Figure 10–3
Sample cover letter responding to an advertised position with bolded areas corresponding to the specifics of the advertisement.

find out as much as possible; if more information is needed, call the employee relations or human resources department and request that this information be sent to you via e-mail, or if it is a local position, you can stop by and pick this information up. Remember to request a position description. Having all this knowledge beforehand will give you added confidence in the interview process.

The preinterview stage can also serve as a practice run-through or stage rehearsal of the actual interview. Here, you can develop answers to questions that are typically asked during the interview process. For example, practice explaining how your skills and experience match the position. The activities at the end of this chapter give you more questions that are often asked so that you can develop a well-thought-out response. Most interviews now follow a **behavioral interview** approach. Employers want to know they are hiring someone who can work well as a team and has the **emotional intelligence (EI)** necessary to make a good fit in the organization. They will ask you questions such as, "Tell me about a time during your clinical practicum when you failed and how you handled that situation" or "Give me a specific example of how you coped with a stressful team situation?" You should try to think of engaging stories from your previous work experience or clinical experiences.

The day of the actual interview has now arrived. A mild level of nervousness and anticipation is to be expected. Your manner of dress and prompt arrival are two very important aspects of the interview process. You should be neat and well groomed with a professional and conservative appearance. Trendy clothes, sneakers, and excessive makeup or jewelry will not impress your potential employer and may even discourage them from considering you, no matter how well the interview goes.

Remember to bring a copy of your résumé and a small notepad and pen. The notepad will allow you to take notes and again show your level of preparedness for the interview. In addition, you may want to have some questions prepared in your notepad to ask at the appropriate time during the interview.

Being late for your interview will send a red flag to the employer concerning your professionalism. Make sure you know exactly where the interview is being held, and plan on arriving early. Make sure you have good directions, and if it is someplace you have never been before, you may want to drive there the day before. Allow for traffic, construction, car problems, or any other unforeseen event. You can always wait in your car or go to the cafeteria or coffee shop once you arrive at the interview site if you are too early. Again, plan on arriving at the interview site at least 10 to 15 minutes early!

While you are waiting to be called in for the interview, make sure you treat the receptionists (and everyone else) with the utmost respect and professionalism. You would be surprised how much of a say they may have in the selection process. When the time comes for the interview and you are called in, remember that you have done your homework and you are prepared. Greet the interviewer(s) with friendliness by introducing yourself and firmly shaking hands. Look each person directly in the eye while speaking to them. Wait to be seated until you are shown your chair, as a sign of respect. Let the interviewer(s) initiate the conversation and follow that person's lead. Everyone interviewing you will be different, and just keep in mind that you are trying to make a good impression as well as learn as much as you can about the position.

Respond to the various interviewers' styles accordingly. Some interviewers may ask very specific questions and expect direct and to-the-point answers. Others may ramble on and want you to do a lot of listening. Still others may ask you open-ended questions such as, "Tell me why you're the person for this position" and expect you to elaborate at length. No matter what the style, you are there to convince them that *you are the best person for the position.* Some "don'ts" of the interview process that can hamper your chance of success include the following:

Top 10 List of Things *Not* to Do at an Interview

- Do not criticize, complain, or blame others (especially former employers).
- Do not exhibit nervous or unprofessional habits such as chewing gum, eating candy, checking your cell phone, or smoking.
- Do not interrupt.
- Do not use slang or nonstandard English.
- Do not discuss controversial topics such as politics or religion.
- Do not discuss your financial or personal problems.
- Do not lie.
- Do not be disrespectful or sarcastic.
- Do not daydream or lose your focus.
- Do not forget to be friendly and open and to show your enthusiasm.

Your job is not done after the interview. The *post interview stage* is also critical. Here you will follow up appropriately and continue to demonstrate your professionalism as well as your interest in the position. Your follow-up should include a brief thank-you letter for the interviewer's time and consideration. Even if you do not get the position, this will leave a favorable impression for future opportunities. Besides, it is the right thing to do. These authors believe that the best thank you is a personalized handwritten note on professional stationary; however, a typed correspondence or e-mail is also acceptable practice.

Each interview you attend provides a unique opportunity to critique your performance. What did you do well? In what areas can you improve? Take advantage of each interview as a learning process in sharpening your skills for the future. Do not get discouraged. It may take several interviews to get your first offer. Then again, you may be flooded with offers and have the "nice problem" of choosing the best one.

Just For FUN 10-1

What Would You Say?

Here are some commonly asked standard interview questions. How would you answer them?

1. What are your strengths? _____

2. What are your weaknesses? _____

3. Why should we hire you? _____

4. Where do you see yourself 5 years from now? _____

5. Did you receive any scholarships and academic awards? _____

6. How did you prepare for this interview? _____

7. How do you plan to maintain your competency and remain current within your profession? _____

8. How do you handle difficult people? _____

9. What type of community and committee service have you performed? _____

10. How do you feel about change? _____

Skill Application 10-5 The Interview

Working together in small groups, take turns being the interviewer and the interviewee. Have a third student critique the interviewee or, if possible, videotape the interview process and let everyone critique the performance. Videotaping and viewing yourself perform can identify weak areas such as nervous habits that you may not even be aware you do.

List five areas you will work on to improve from your evaluations of your interview process.

a. _____

b. _____

c. _____

d. _____

e. _____

Your First Career Position: First and Lasting Impressions

There are several impressions you want your employer, coworkers, and patients to have concerning your ability to do your job. You want everyone to know that you take pride in your career and that you are a professional. A health care professional has several characteristics, including commitment to quality work, dependability, and a high level of interpersonal skills.

Commitment to High-Quality Work

The patient/client represents the consumer of health care services. Although we do not want people to become ill, this is a fact of life. Our job is to prevent and treat illness by providing high-quality services. Quality is important for several reasons. First, the quality of our services directly affects the outcomes of the diagnosis or treatment. Second, the quality of our work increases our individual reputation as well as that of the organization. This in turn results in more repeat and referred customers seeking our services. Without patients, health care systems cannot survive and your position is threatened. In addition, lawsuits can flourish and human life suffer when quality of care is poor. Therefore, it is imperative that you strive for high-quality patient care—for the patient's and the organization's sake.

Quality can best be achieved by doing those things that will make you the best possible health care professional you can be. You can be "the best" by learning all you can about your profession. Reading journals, attending seminars, performing continuing medical education, and researching topics will all help you deliver high-quality care because you will be able to use the most current knowledge and techniques.

Dependability

Your patients, coworkers, and supervisors need to know that they can count on you to be there. "Being there" in health care can literally mean the difference between life and death. Therefore, it is important to maintain good attendance and punctuality in your position. A good attendance record shows that you are dependable and can be counted on to be there unless a personal emergency or illness occurs. This characteristic allows other members of the health care team to have faith in your commitment. Good attendance also allows for better continuity of care. If members of the team are habitually absent, information is not passed on well and different levels of care may be given.

Punctuality, or being on time at the start of your shift, is especially important in health care. The start of your shift is when the report from the previous shift is given. This report includes vital information concerning your patients' status and their upcoming treatment schedules. In addition, any unusual circumstances or trends can be relayed at this time. For example, it would be highly beneficial to know that the condition of your patient in room 603 is worsening and that the patient had a tachycardia episode during the administration of the last treatment.

Unforeseen things happen in everyone's life, and there comes a time when you will be absent or late. When this occurs, handle the situation in a professional manner. If you know that you are going to be absent or late, make sure your supervisor knows as soon as possible. For example, if you are sick and know you will not make it to work, call as soon as possible (preferably the day before) so that proper arrangements can be made to cover your shift. If you are going to be late, again, call as soon as possible and give your approximate time of arrival.

It is also important to be punctual on the job. If you are a member of the trauma or code team, it is vital you arrive ASAP (as soon as possible), or as they say in medicine STAT, when a trauma or code is in progress. In addition, punctuality must be maintained on a patient's treatment schedule. Although this may not always be possible, the patient should be notified when there will be changes in the scheduled treatments or tests.

High Level of Interpersonal Skills

In health care, you must be able to have a positive relationship with your patients and coworkers to deliver effective and high-quality care. This type of relationship can be established by incorporating those attitudes and actions that will lead to a positive outcome. The list of ingredients that leads to a positive relationship include the following:

- Competency
- Trust
- Empathy
- Respect
- Ability to give and receive feedback

Competency refers to your ability to do your job well. In other words, do you "know your stuff"? This requires you to take pride in your professional career both while in training and after you graduate. You must continue to be a lifelong learner in the health care profession because the advancement of new knowledge and techniques occurs continuously. Competency also requires you to have self-confidence. Even if you "know your stuff," if you doubt your abilities, the patient will perceive you as not competent. In addition, a confident (not arrogant) attitude will be respected by other members of the health care team.

Test Yourself 10–1

Do You Have What It Takes?

Picture yourself on the job. Drawing from your past work and life experiences, how would you rate yourself in the following areas? Fill in the blanks with *Expert* (no work needed), *Novice* (need improvement), or *Beginner* (need to really work on this area).

1. _____ I am committed to quality and doing the best job I possibly can with every aspect of the job, even the dull and tedious tasks.

2. _____ I am highly dependable and can be counted on to always be there.

3. _____ I am always on time (or even a little early) when reporting for work or meeting with someone.

4. _____ I am constantly learning about my profession and learning new information and techniques to remain highly competent.

5. _____ I can always be trusted with confidential information.

6. _____ I can empathize with others.

7. _____ I respect the rights and beliefs of all individuals, even those I do not agree with.

This is a test in which the authors feel you should have no *Expert* answers. We can all improve our skills in these areas (even the authors) and should continually strive to do so.

Any good relationship is based on **trust**. Trust means that you can be relied on to get the job done well and maintain professional standards such as ethics and confidentiality. Trust is hard to get but easy to lose. It must be based on consistent behavior that demonstrates that your patients and coworkers can trust you with confidential information.

Respect means that you value your patients and coworkers. Respect is shown by being courteous and understanding in even the most difficult situations. Related to respect is **empathy**. Empathy is the ability to "feel what others are going through." An old phrase states not to judge people until you have "walked a mile in their shoes." Empathy allows us to understand what at times may appear to be irrational behavior.

Positive interpersonal relationships also require *feedback* to occur. It is important to learn to give and get feedback from your patients and their families as well as from your coworkers. Feedback makes relationships grow and develop. Positive feedback such as praise for a job well done is easy to give and appreciated by the receiver. However, sometimes feedback is negative, which is harder to give and receive.

Feedback should always be given in a nonthreatening manner. The goal of all feedback (even negative) should be to help the other person. Remember, the person who is giving or receiving feedback should always feel respected and valued. General rules concerning feedback include the following:

- Praise publicly and criticize privately.
- Your motivation with all feedback should be to help the other person.
- Resist judging others when giving feedback.
- Criticize specific behavior and not the individual personally.

Skill Application 10–6 Impressions on the Job

For each word or phrase listed, give a brief explanation of what it means to you personally. Then, write a sentence on how it will relate to you in your first position in health care.

1. Commitment to quality work

   Personal meaning: _____

   How does it relate to my first position in health care? _____

2. Dependability

   Personal meaning: _____

   How does it relate to my first position in health care? _____

3. Punctuality

   Personal meaning: _____

   How does it relate to my first position in health care? _____

4. Empathy

   Personal meaning: _____

   How does it relate to my first position in health care? _____

5. Trust

   Personal meaning: _____

   How does it relate to my first position in health care? _____

6. Respect

   Personal meaning: _____

   How does it relate to my first position in health care? _____

(continues)

(continued)

Feedback

1. Give an example of when you handled negative feedback appropriately.

_____

2. Give an example of when you did not handle feedback appropriately.

_____

The Importance of Professional Image

Food for Thought 10–1

Great Minds Think Alike

We make a living by what we get, but we make a life by what we give.

—Winston Churchill

Suppose you were asked to interpret this quote during a job interview. How would you respond? What personal examples could you offer to illustrate your understanding of this quote?

You are now about to embark on your chosen professional career in health care. Your respective profession is counting on you to represent it in a positive manner to your patients, coworkers, and employer. Joining your professional organization is a very important step in the further development of your **professional image**, showcasing yourself and career.

Professional image affects the number and quality of persons choosing a certain profession. A high professional image means that more high-quality individuals will choose the profession you represent, which in turn will keep the standards high.

Public opinion is vital to the success of any profession. A positive image affects the outcome of treatments and enhances your interaction with patients. A positive image also lends credence to your interaction with other health care professionals. You can contribute to your professional image by becoming an active member of your professional organization.

Methods to Improve Professional Image

The best method for enhancing professional image is to demonstrate that you have the expert knowledge in your field. This can be shown by your competency levels when performing your job, your willingness to learn new procedures, and your continual pursuit of lifelong learning. Reading journals and attending seminars and in-services will lend to this image. The more you know about your profession and your area of expertise, the more difficult it will be to replace you. Therefore, this knowledge relates directly to your job security.

At work always strive to increase your visibility in a positive way. Offer to do in-services and train others both within your department and from other areas. Teaching other health care professionals about your area by providing in-service programs to other departments shows your knowledge, openness, and ability to work as a team member. This helps build camaraderie and mutual respect.

Get involved in health care committees to help network and represent yourself and your profession within the organization. Cooperation with other professionals will maintain an open system of communication and allow your talents to be fully realized. Good luck on your health professional career. You will touch the lives of many people.

Skill Application 10–7 **Researching Your Profession**

Learning about your chosen profession is the first important step in achieving a positive professional image. Go to the website of the national headquarters for your profession and obtain as much information as you can to answer the following:

1. Name of profession: _____

2. Headquarters' address and telephone numbers: _____

3. Profession description: _____

4. Professional credentials: _____

5. Professional publications: _____

6. Requirements for licensing if applicable: _____

7. Continuing education requirements: _____

Summary

- Remember to always strive to showcase your high-quality professional image.

- You have worked hard to graduate from your chosen school and become a professional. However, the work is not done. You must now either decide on more education or look for your first position (in some cases both). Regardless of the path you choose, the potential rewards can be great. These rewards go beyond monetary compensation and include a chance to really make a difference to others' health and lives.

- Your first job in health care will be quite rewarding. However, to make sure that you secure the best position for yourself, you must perform several preparatory steps.

- The first step is analyzing the type of position you want.
- You will then proceed to develop a professional résumé and make initial contacts and find position openings.
- A professional cover letter will assist you in getting to the interview stage.
- Extensive preparation and practice before your interview will enhance your performance and optimize your chance of getting the position.
- Once you have secured a position, you must continue to grow and develop in your new profession. You must demonstrate a commitment to high-quality work, dependability, and good interpersonal skills.

- You must maintain competency by continuing the learning process and maintaining current knowledge about new advances in your chosen practice.
- The pursuit of your first position requires careful preparation and planning. This chapter helped you prepare for your quest in finding the position that is right for you. In addition, this chapter conveys the importance of a professional image and lifelong learning. Remember, a health care professional is truly a unique individual. This field requires you to become a lifelong learner in order to maintain competency and stay current within your profession.

Case Study 10–1

Tara Smith worked as a dental technician in the office for almost 4 years. Tara was a dependable employee and performed adequately with good technical skills. She made to not keep up with advances in her field by attending seminars or conferences or volunteer for special projects. She was never rude to her patients but gave the impression she was simply doing her job and anxious to finish her shift. Tara was very surprised and upset when a coworker who was only in the office for a little over a year was chosen for a promotion and Tara was not. Is Tara's disappointment justified? Describe some of the things Tara could have done differently in order to put herself in a better position to get future promotions.

_____

_____

Internet Activity

Using Internet search engines, find additional material on "your first position as a health care professional" that can help you and your fellow students. Some suggested keywords are job searching, résumé writing, cover letters, interviewing skills, and professional image. Write down something new that you found to share.

_____

_____

Chapter 11

Professionalism in Action

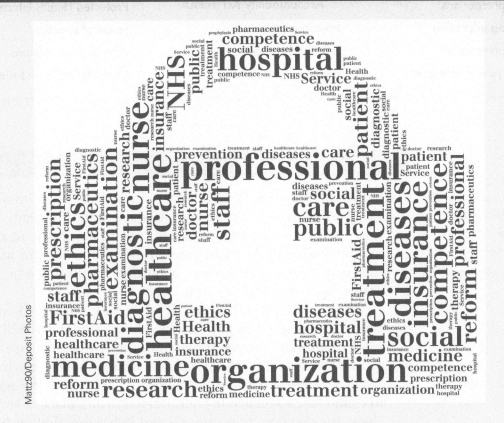

Mattz90/Deposit Photos

Objectives

Upon completion of this chapter, you should be able to:

1. Examine ethical issues that include confidentiality, respect, trust, death and dying, and euthanasia.

2. Explain infection control measures to protect both yourself and your patient.

3. Examine medical-legal issues that include malpractice, negligence, the patient's rights, and infection control.

4. Examine aspects that enhance the patient care partnership with both the health professional and the health care institution.

Key Terms

advanced directive	ethics	malpractice
against medical advice (AMA)	euthanasia	negligence
airborne precautions	health care proxy	palliative care
certification	Health Insurance Portability and	personal protective equipment (PPE)
contact precautions	Accountability Act (HIPAA)	Protected Health Information (PHI)
continuing education	hospice care	scope of practice
droplet precautions	informed consent	standard precautions
durable power of attorney	living will	transmission-based precautions

Introduction

The real voyage of discovery rests not in seeking new landscapes, but in having new eyes.

—Marcel Proust

This final chapter will help assist you with the key ingredients for a successful career. At the end of your successful graduation from your health care program, you will obtain employment as a health care professional. As such, you will be responsible for maintaining your license and certification, obtaining continuing education, and staying up to date on current issues.

Additionally, this chapter will take a look at many common issues that face all heath care professions. There is great variability in what will be required between professions and within the areas in which you are employed; there are common threads however, which will be discussed here. Ultimately, you will be responsible for maintaining all competencies related to your profession and place of employment. There are also common professional behaviors that all health care professionals should engage in; some examples include behaving in an ethical manner, showing respect, understanding the legal issues related to health care, and providing excellent customer service.

Anticipatory Exercise 11–1 Code of Ethics

Go to the Internet and find the American Medical Association's Code of Medical Ethics. Review the Web page, and list three of the principles that you would like more information about. Take some time to look for more information on the topics you chose.

1. _____

2. _____

3. _____

Medical Ethics

Ethical decision-making arises almost daily in all areas of health care. You will have access to confidential information concerning many aspects of a person's life. In addition, you are ethically bound to be current and competent with the level of care you will be administering to your patients. All health care professionals should familiarize themselves with and practice the stated code of ethics related to their profession. Health care professionals must also familiarize themselves with legal issues such as malpractice, negligence, and scope of practice.

Ethics is defined in dictionaries as moral principles or practices. In life, it means knowing the difference between right and wrong. In health care, it means conforming to accepted and professional standards of conduct. In both life and health care, ethical behavior is "doing the right thing in the right way." Ethics should govern and guide the way you act and the proper decisions you make. There are several situations in which ethics will influence decisions about patient care. These areas include confidentiality, respect, trust, and death and dying.

Confidentiality

Confidentiality means keeping information private and not sharing it with inappropriate people. You will have access to information concerning your patient that includes diagnosis, medical history, and lifestyle. You can discuss this information only with other health care professionals who are caring for this patient. You must use discretion when discussing patient information. Figure 11–1 shows some of the confidential information you may have access to in a medical chart.

For example, you may be in the cafeteria and say something as innocent such as, "I feel so bad for Mr. Smith in 408, his cancer biopsy was positive." Mr. Smith's family may be seated next to you and hear what you said. They may not know this information yet, and although you meant no harm, you have acted in an unprofessional and unethical manner.

One other aspect of confidentiality is that it is the physician's responsibility to tell the patient the results of tests or the diagnosis. You should discuss only the information related to the therapy or intervention you are performing.

MEDICAL HISTORY FORM

Date _____
Patient's name _____

Age	Date of birth	Sex

Address	City	State	Zip code

Phone ( )

Insurance company	Policy number

Place of employment	Address

Phone ( )	Job responsibilities

Parent/Guardian if minor

Address	City	State	Zip code

Phone ( )

Family History:

List family members: (mother, father, brothers, sisters, grandparents, etc.)—ages and health status (if deceased write their age at the time of their death and the cause). List allergies and/or any conditions or diseases they may have or have had, such as asthma, arthritis, tuberculosis, diabetes, cancer, heart disease, hypertension, kidney disease, mental illness, depression, or any other health problems that you know of in your family.

_____

_____

Patient's Past History: Mark the boxes to the right either "yes" or "no" for the following questions:*

Do you ever have or have you ever had any of the following: **(yes) (no)**

SKIN
Rashes, hives, itching or other skin irritations ( ) ( )

EYES, EARS, NOSE, THROAT
Headaches, dizziness, fainting ( ) ( )
Blurred or impaired vision ( ) ( )
Hearing loss or ringing in the ears ( ) ( )
Discharge from eyes or ears ( ) ( )
Sinus trouble/colds/allergies ( ) ( )
Asthma or hay fever ( ) ( )
Sore throats/hoarseness ( ) ( )

CARDIOPULMONARY
Shortness of breath ( ) ( )
Persistent cough or coughing up blood or other secretions ( ) ( )
Chills and/or fever ( ) ( )
Night sweats ( ) ( )
Tuberculosis or exposed to TB ( ) ( )

Scarlet fever or rheumatic fever ( ) ( )
Chest pain ( ) ( )
Heart palpitations or rapid heartbeat or pulse ( ) ( )
High blood pressure ( ) ( )
Swelling of hands and/or feet ( ) ( )

GASTROINTESTINAL
Heartburn or indigestion ( ) ( )
Nausea and/or vomiting ( ) ( )
Loss of appetite ( ) ( )
Belching or gas ( ) ( )
Peptic ulcer, gallbladder or liver disease ( ) ( )
Yellow jaundice or hepatitis ( ) ( )
Diarrhea or constipation ( ) ( )
Dysentery ( ) ( )
Rectal bleeding, hemorrhoids (piles) ( ) ( )
Tarry or clay-colored stools ( ) ( )

GLANDS
Weight gain or loss ( ) ( )

Diabetes ( ) ( )
Thyroid or goiter ( ) ( )
Swollen glands ( ) ( )

GENITOURINARY
Kidney disease or stones, or Bright's disease ( ) ( )
Painful, frequent or urgent urination ( ) ( )
Blood or pus in urine ( ) ( )
Sexually transmitted disease (venereal disease) ( ) ( )
Been sexually active with anyone who has AIDS or HIV or hepatitis ( ) ( )

NEUROMUSCULAR
Problems with becoming tired and/or upset easily ( ) ( )
Nervous breakdown/depression ( ) ( )
Poliomyelitis (infantile paralysis) ( ) ( )
Convulsions ( ) ( )
Joint and/or muscular pain ( ) ( )
Back pain or injury/osteomyelitis/rheumatism ( ) ( )

Are you currently taking any medications? **Yes ( ) No ( )**
If yes, please list them _____
Have you ever had or been treated for cancer or any tumors? ( ) ( )
Are you anemic or have you ever had to take iron medication? ( ) ( )
Do you use tobacco? ( ) ( )
What type? _____
Do you use IV drugs or alcohol? ( ) ( )

WOMEN ONLY
Painful menstrual periods ( ) ( )
Pregnancy/abortion/miscarriage ( ) ( )
Vaginal infection or discharge/abnormal bleeding ( ) ( )

Last menstrual period _____
Birth control _____
List dates of all operations/surgeries, injuries, and illnesses that required hospitalization:
_____
_____

Did you ever receive benefits from a medical insurance claim due to illness or injury? **Yes ( ) No ( )**
Were you ever rejected from the military or for employment? ( ) ( )
Were you absent from school/work in the past 10 years because of illness or injury? ( ) ( )
Did you ever file a Workers' Compensation claim? ( ) ( )
Did you ever seek psychological or psychiatric treatment? ( ) ( )

*Please use the back of this form to explain any "yes" answers. Thank you.

Figure 11–1
A sample of some of the confidential information to which you will have access in the medical record.

Food for Thought 11–1

Confidential Issues

What is wrong with the following situations?

1. You go home and tell one of your friends that you gave therapy to their cousin in the hospital today.

2. You tell someone at a party how surprised you were to find out that a patient you both know was diagnosed with an alcohol use disorder.

3. You discuss a patient's past medical history or illness with another health care professional who is not involved in the case.

4. You tell a patient that they do not have the "bad" kind of cancer.

Respect

Each person deserves to be shown respect during the course of treatment. You may not agree with a patient's religious beliefs or choice of lifestyle, but again they may not agree with yours. Health care professionals are not to be judgmental. Your job is to deliver appropriate and considerate therapy to *all* your patients.

You will also encounter difficult patients who may be hostile, angry, or withdrawn. They may upset you with their actions, words, or refusal to comply with therapies. It is important to remember there are no professional patients; they are all experiencing a stressful situation that typically is not of their choosing. Again, you must respect their situation and place yourself in their shoes (or in this case hospital gown) and show them empathy. They probably have good reason for their mood. You should remain calm and not argue with them. Arguing will only worsen the situation. Calmness and consistent, considerate care will usually help the patient's demeanor and aid in compliance with therapy.

Trust

Trust is an important ethical ingredient. A patient who trusts the health care professional will be more cooperative with the therapy and more forthcoming with information. Trust can be developed in several ways. First, you should be careful in handling the patient's personal belongings. You should follow your organization's policy and procedure in this matter. For example, most organizations require that a health care worker complete a checklist that lists the belongings of the patients while in the hospital.

Patients trust you to be dependable and meet their needs in a timely fashion (i.e., have their therapy, bath, and food tray on time). This enhances trusting relationships. If a situation arises in which the schedule cannot be met, the circumstances should be explained to the patient.

Patients also trust that they will be safe and protected from harm. For example, patients often need transportation to other areas within the hospital. If certain rules are not followed, patient transport can be potentially dangerous. You need to make sure you know and follow your institution's safety guidelines for patient transport. For example, one common rule is to lock the wheels of transport devices such as stretchers (the moving beds) and wheelchairs when they are not moving. Can you imagine what would happen if an unattended patient in an unlocked wheelchair fell down a flight of steps?

Another way to protect the patient from harm is to report any suspected abuse. By law, health care professionals must report any abuse of a person under 18 years of age. This is because as health care professionals we are mandated reporters of any suspected abuse of children. However, you should report all cases, regardless of age, to the proper person. In many cases, the proper person is the nurse in charge of that area or the social service department.

Abuse can take on four specific forms. *Physical abuse* results from actual contact, usually resulting in a visible injury. Although physical abuse can sometimes be evident by bruise marks on the patient, neglect such as not feeding or providing a safe environment can also be classified as physical abuse.

Verbal abuse occurs when spoken words are meant to hurt another person's self-esteem. This can make a person feel unimportant, worthless, or bad about themselves.

Psychological abuse is sometimes harder to see or hear. This abuse results in a fearful state for the person being abused. This can take the form of vicious threats such as, "If you wet the bed one more time, I'll let you sleep in it."

Sexual abuse is any inappropriate sexual touch or act. As a health care practitioner, you will be in a position of authority over patients. This authority comes from your expert knowledge. The practitioner–patient relationship gives you control over many situations. Add to this the fact that patients are often in very vulnerable states and you could have the potential for sexual abuse. Therefore, sexual relations with patients are unethical and would interfere with the therapeutic relationship that should exist between a practitioner and patient.

Elder abuse is the mistreatment of older adults. As people age they tend to become more dependent on others, putting them at risk for abuse. Elder abuse can include any of the types of abuse discussed previously, plus several other forms. Removal of decision-making power from older adults who are still competent, neglect in providing basic necessities, and financial exploitation are additional forms of abuse that older adults may experience. It is the health care professionals' responsibility to report suspected elder abuse.

Food for Thought 11–2

Sources of Abuse

Abuse can come from family members, friends, or complete strangers. However, abuse can also be caused by health care professionals. Can you think of examples of when health care professionals could abuse their patients? What would you do if you witnessed abuse?

Skill Application 11–1 Ethical and Unethical Situations

Provide an example of an ethical and unethical situation for each of the categories. They may be from your past professional or personal experiences or from something you have heard or seen in the media.

1. **Confidentiality**

   Ethical situation: _____

   _____

   _____

   Unethical situation: _____

   _____

   _____

2. **Respect**

   Ethical situation: _____

   _____

   _____

   Unethical situation: _____

   _____

   _____

3. **Trust**

   Ethical situation: _____

   _____

   _____

   Unethical situation: _____

   _____

   _____

Death and Dying

Death and dying is an ethical issue we must all face. As health care professionals, we will deal with this issue on a more frequent basis. Not only may we witness death occur during a cardiac or respiratory arrest, but we will also experience the process of dying through our terminally ill patients. Therefore, it is important to examine many of your own feelings and beliefs concerning death and dying. The first step is to understand what usually occurs during the process of dying. Dr. Elizabeth Kübler-Ross did a great deal of work with patients dying of terminal illness. Her extensive study led to the identification of the following five stages of grieving that occurs during the dying process:

- Denial
- Anger
- Bargaining
- Depression
- Acceptance

Denial, usually the first stage of the grieving process, occurs after the patient is made aware of the terminal diagnosis. Here, the patient denies having the disease with statements such as, "The tests must be wrong" or "It can't be that bad."

The second stage, *anger*, usually follows denial, and the patient becomes hostile and bitter about the situation. The health care professional may become the target of the patient's anger. Remember, do not take any anger directed at you personally. It is best to be supportive and understanding with the patient at all times.

The third stage identified is *bargaining*. During this stage, the patient bargains according to their spiritual beliefs. The patient may plead, "Please let me live to see my grandchild." Again, your best response is to actively listen and provide support.

Depression represents the fourth stage of the grieving process. This is usually when the patient becomes withdrawn and extremely sad. The patient may break down and cry. Again, your support is what is needed. You may even find yourself getting emotional with the patient, and a gentle touch at the appropriate time may help.

The fifth and final stage is *acceptance*. At this time, the patient will want to complete unfinished business, and your support in facilitating this is important. A certain calm may be experienced by the patient during this stage.

Patients may move through these stages in different orders; however, you can usually identify what stage they are in by their moods, actions, and language used (see Figure 11–2). Understanding the stages will also help you cope with their death. For example, you may have a patient you have come to know very well over time. After being diagnosed as having a terminal disease, the patient may become angry or withdraw from you. It is important that you understand that this

Figure 11–2
Verbal examples of
the stages of death
and dying.

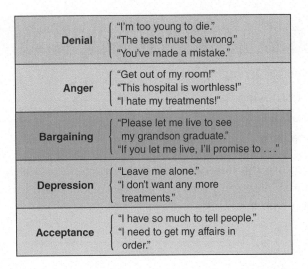

Denial	"I'm too young to die." "The tests must be wrong." "You've made a mistake."
Anger	"Get out of my room!" "This hospital is worthless!" "I hate my treatments!"
Bargaining	"Please let me live to see my grandson graduate." "If you let me live, I'll promise to . . ."
Depression	"Leave me alone." "I don't want any more treatments."
Acceptance	"I have so much to tell people." "I need to get my affairs in order."

is a normal part of the grieving process and not personally directed at you. You will also see those who care for the patient (family and friends) going through the stages of grief, especially after the patient dies. After a patient dies, the family becomes your new patient.

There are special parts of the health care system that care for patient with terminal illness; they are **palliative care** and **hospice care**. These two types of care are similar, yet have some distinctions. Hospice is not a place but a type of care that helps the patient and family throughout the grieving process and allows the patient to die with dignity, usually at home where the patient feels most comfortable. Hospice care is for those at the end of a terminal illness, or when they are no longer seeking curative care. Palliative care provides care for those facing life-threatening illness, at any point in the illness. This type of care is provided by a team of health care providers and seeks to improve quality of life, relieve suffering, and support the patient and family in navigating the medical system.

There are also parts of the health care system called long-term acute care (LTAC) that care for chronically critically ill patients. These may be patients who have chronic tracheostomy tubes, severe wounds, or brain injuries such as stroke or trauma. These LTACs use evidence-based treatments over the course of approximately 30 days to help the patient progress through their illness to the next level of care.

Inpatient rehabilitation facilities provide therapies to patients including occupational, physical, and speech language. Patients must be able to participate in 3 hours of therapy each day to be able to qualify for admission. The goal of inpatient rehabilitation is to return the patient to their previous living arrangement.

Any of these health care facilities are not the first stop in a long duration of navigating the health care system. Patients and families who experience illness have many needs and stresses that can be supported by qualified and compassionate health care providers such as yourself.

Skill Application 11–2 Ethical Issues

Research the following topics:

- Death and dying
- Euthanasia
- Hospice care

You can use the Internet or library, or you can call a local hospice unit. In one paragraph, write the most interesting fact you learned about these topics that was not included in this chapter, and share it with the class.

1. Death and dying: _____

   _____

   _____

   _____

2. Euthanasia: _____

   _____

   _____

   _____

3. Hospice care: _____

   _____

   _____

   _____

Euthanasia

The right to die is a controversial issue. **Euthanasia** technically means an "easy death." In health care, it is the concept of medically assisting another to die. Euthanasia can be divided into a passive or active form. Passive euthanasia is the process of withholding treatment that could sustain a life. Active euthanasia is actively assisting the patient in dying.

The question arises whether advanced life support should be withheld or withdrawn from certain terminally ill patients. Although death is a natural progression of life, there are still many questions about just what death is. *Brain death* is defined as the irreversible cessation of all functions of the brain. This state goes beyond a coma-tose (coma) state in which the brain is still functioning to maintain life and the patient still has the ability for conscious thought.

With advances in technology, life support equipment can maintain someone's life who is brain dead for months and even years.

This state of being is called a *persistent vegetative state*; the patient is in a permanent state of unconsciousness, and the vital functions of the body are performed by machines.

Many would argue that someone in a persistent vegetative state is really not alive. This raises the question of one's quality of life. The quality of life looks at the individual's potential ability to return to a conscious state and function at a level that maintains qualities such as awareness and human interaction. People who believe in the quality of life issues believe the major goal of health care should be to maintain the quality of life of the individual.

Food for Thought 11–3

Mercy Killing
Active voluntary euthanasia can be termed mercy killing. What are your thoughts concerning this concept? Can you find any recent news articles related to this concept?

Food for Thought 11–4

Above and Beyond the Call?
Depending on the physician's beliefs, treatments can take various forms. For example, physicians who believe all measures should be taken at all times to continue life will use extraordinary means. Extraordinary means include using all medicines, treatments, and operations, regardless of expense, pain, or other inconveniences to patient or family. What do you think about extraordinary care? Should expense be a consideration?

Skill Application 11–3 Ethical Debates

Pair off in groups of four to six. Choose an ethical topic to debate. For example, is physician-assisted death justifiable? If so, under what circumstances? Your group should develop an ethical dilemma or question and then debate the issue and list the various viewpoints. Remember, there are no clear right or wrong answers, and you should listen to the differing viewpoints of others with respect.

Your group's ethical dilemma or question: _____

_____

_____

_____

(continues)

(continued)

Various viewpoints: _____

_____

_____

_____

_____

Food for Thought 11–5

What Do You Believe?

Ponder your personal beliefs given the following questions:

When does life begin? When does life end?

How would you define quality of life?

Is assisted death justified?

Should organs of a person who is brain dead be harvested and used to save other lives?

Infection Control

To help protect the health of your patients, coworkers, and yourself, you need to have a basic understanding of *infection control*. Infection control includes policies and procedures regarding transmission of communicable diseases. The *chain of infection* begins with a source of infection, continues with the transportation of the infection, and ends with the entry into the body (see Figure 11–3).

Pathogens find their way inside of us and cause infections through various *routes of transmission*. These routes include contact (direct or indirect), common vehicle, airborne, and vector

Figure 11–3
An illustration of the chain of infection.

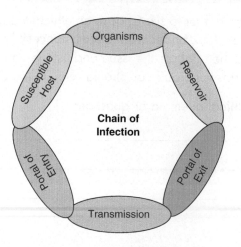

(biological or mechanical) routes of transmission. To help health care professionals protect themselves and other patients from the spread of infection, the Centers for Disease Control and Prevention (CDC) and the Occupational Safety and Health Administration (OSHA) have developed isolation precautions to help create barriers between people and germs. There are two types of isolation precautions: **standard precautions** and **transmission-based precautions**. Standard precautions should be followed for all patients. The standard precaution guidelines state that when you are close to or touching blood, body fluid, body tissues, mucous membranes, or other open skin areas, you must use hand hygiene and **personal protective equipment (PPE)**. The PPE includes gloves, masks, goggles, apron, gowns, and shoe covers. How many of these items you wear depend on what type of interaction or intervention you will be encountering. The PPE equipment must be provided by your employer per regulations set forth by the OSHA. Figure 11–4 depicts a health care professional wearing PPE.

Transmission-based precautions can be further broken down into three subcategories: **airborne precautions**, **contact precautions**, and **droplet precautions**. These transmission-based precautions are in addition to the standard precaution and are utilized based on confirmed or suspected diagnosis. Airborne precautions are needed for germs that are so small they can float in the air (an example is tuberculosis). Patients on airborne precautions are placed in a special *negative pressure room* and anyone caring for these patients must wear a special custom-fit respirator mask. Contact precautions are needed for germs

Figure 11–4
A health care provider wearing personal protective equipment (PPE).

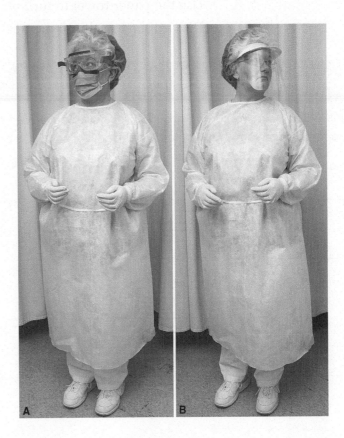

that spread by touch or contact (an example is *Clostridioides difficile*). Any person or visitor entering a contact precaution room must wear gloves and a gown. Droplet precautions are used for those patients who have a disease that is spread through secretions from the nose, sinuses, throat, airways, and lungs (an example is influenza). Everyone who enters a room with droplet precautions should wear a surgical mask.

No matter what diagnosis or type of illness the patient has, the goal is to prevent the spread of infection to yourself, family, or other patients by breaking the chain of infection at some point along the way. The single most effective way to break the chain of infection is through *hand washing* or *hand hygiene*. Hand washing should be done after touching blood, body fluids, secretions, excretions, and contaminated items. Wash before applying gloves and after removing them and always between patient contacts. There is a proper way to wash your hands:

- Remove all jewelry from your hands.
- Crank out enough paper towel to dry your hands but do not tear it off.
- Turn on the water as hot as tolerable.
- Wet hands and apply soap.
- Work the soapy water over your hands, between fingers, and around nails.
- Continue this action for at least 25 to 30 seconds.
- Rinse with water, positioning your hands so the water flows from above the wrists, downward and over the hands, and then fingers.
- Tear off the paper towel, and dry hands.
- Use the paper towel to turn off the water.
- Discard the towel into the trash can.

Skill Application 11–4 Infection Control

Either individually or working in groups, develop a case scenario concerning infection control and describe the precautions that would be needed. Appendix B can give you some useful information.

Scenario:

_____

_____

_____

Infection control measures required:

_____

_____

_____

_____

Legal Issues

The patient's well-being is entrusted to the various health care practitioners providing care. Each state has written laws or statutes that define what certified or licensed health care workers can do. This is called the **scope of practice**. You cannot exceed your scope of practice because this is what you were specifically trained to do and legally allowed to do. State boards regulate the licensee or certificate holder and can revoke the license for violation of scope of practice or involvement in other stated offenses such as drug abuse, sexual abuse, felonies, and so on.

In addition to a defined scope of practice, each health care organization has its own guidelines and established ways of doing things. These guidelines can take the form of policies, procedures, and protocols. *Protocols* help standardize care and help establish "how and when to do your specific procedures and interventions" in specific situations. For example, a patient safety protocol may state that all side rails must be raised when transporting a patient on a stretcher. Another protocol you may be familiar with is that of basic life support or cardiopulmonary resuscitation (CPR). Figure 11–5 shows the survival chain CPR protocol.

Negligence and Malpractice

Two general types of legal actions can be taken against a health care worker in the line of duty: **negligence** and **malpractice**. Negligence is the failure to give reasonable care and can be intentional or unintentional. Intentional negligence includes battery, false imprisonment, abandonment, invasion of privacy, and fraud. Some examples of unintentional negligence are forgetting to put the side rails up or not immediately cleaning up a spill. The medical term *mal* means bad. Therefore, malpractice can be thought of as bad practice. Malpractice is any professional misconduct or lack of competency that results in injury to the patient. Performing a procedure incorrectly or practicing outside your scope of practice or competency level constitutes malpractice.

Battery means using touch or force without the patient's consent. This includes doing a procedure without having the patient's proper consent. Each patient has the right to determine what can and cannot be done. All health care facilities should have a consent form that the patient must sign before admission and certain procedures. Any type of surgical procedure requires an **informed consent**. Informed means that the patient has been instructed about what the procedure entails. All consents require a witness 21 years of age or older and should be signed in black ink. Consents can be given over the telephone in certain situations. Accepting telephone consent requires two people to listen at the same time.

Figure 11–5
CPR survival chain protocol.

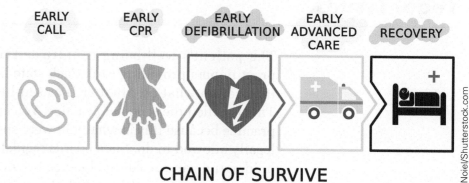

CHAIN OF SURVIVE

Other Legal Issues

False imprisonment is restraining a person against their will. Sometimes it may be necessary to use restraining measures to prevent patients from doing harm to themselves or others. However, one should not restrain a patient because they are being difficult or because it would make the health care professional's job easier. In health care, a physician order is required to restrain any patient. Some patients may insist on leaving the health care institution, even when it may not be in their best interest. If a patient insists on leaving, they may be signed out "**against medical advice**" (AMA), meaning that a health care professional has advised the patient against leaving and has explained the possible dangers of disrupting treatment.

Abandonment is leaving a patient who needs additional care. For example, you notice a patient is drowning in their own secretions and you simply leave the room instead of clearing the secretions. This is a form of abandonment.

Invasion of privacy is any public discussion of private information concerning your patient. This includes discussing a diagnosis, biographical information, and lifestyle preferences. Because you have access to privileged information, you must always maintain confidentiality. Follow the rule to discuss patient issues only with other health care professionals, and then only when that discussion adds to the treatment of the patient.

Invasion of privacy also includes the patient's body being handled by someone not involved in care or the patient's personal belongings being handled without permission. Protect your patients' privacy by knocking before entering a room, drawing curtains while performing procedures, and protecting them from exposure from hospital gowns. In addition, allow visitors time alone with the patient, and do not listen to conversations and telephone calls.

Privacy is such an important issue that federal legislation was enacted to further protect the confidentiality of medical records and information. The **Health Insurance Portability and Accountability**

Act (HIPAA) of 1996 established a well-defined set of regulations concerning protection of patient privacy. This federal legislation covered the following three areas:

1. Insurance Portability: Ensures individuals' ability to maintain health insurance coverage when they switch from one health plan to another. In addition, it prevents health plans from denying coverage due to a preexisting condition.

2. Administrative Simplification: This part of the act requires health care providers and health insurance plans to standardize the process they use to exchange electronic information and implement policies to protect this exchange of information as it relates to patient confidentiality.

3. Privacy and Security: This section of the act requires that health care providers use methods to ensure that a patient's medical information is secure and private.

All health care organizations should have HIPAA policies and training sessions that demonstrate compliance with this important federal legislation. Information about an individual and their health information are considered **Protected Health Information (PHI)** and include the following:

*   Name
*   Medical record number
*   Social Security number
*   Address
*   Date of birth
*   Diagnosis
*   Medical history
*   Medications

Some highlights of policies common to many organizations as a result of HIPAA are as follows:

*   Patients must sign a release before any PHI information can be released.
*   Patients should be made aware of HIPAA, how their information is protected, and whom to contact if they suspect a violation.
*   Patients have a right to access and view their health information in most cases.
*   Patients can request to amend or correct their PHI if they feel it is in error.
*   PHI should only be available to staff on a "need to know in order to do their job" basis.
*   Oral communication is a common breach of confidentiality, and policies should address this also.

- Medical information should be physically (locked) and electronically secured (codes and passwords) to prevent unauthorized access.
- Be careful of photocopies and faxed information others can view.
- Medical information should be properly disposed.

Making sure everyone in your facility is HIPAA compliant not only protects the patients but also the employees and the financial situation of the organization. Violations of HIPAA can result in penalties and fines up to $250,000 and 10 years of imprisonment.

Fraud consists of the intentional withholding or modification of information. For example, modifying a chart to cover up a medication error is a fraudulent act.

 Test Yourself 11–1

Negligence or Malpractice

Negligence and malpractice are often confused. Identify each of the following as an act of negligence or malpractice.

1. Applying a heat pack that burns a patient
2. Performing a procedure that is outside your scope of practice
3. Restraining a patient because you are tired of them pulling out the intravenous line
4. Performing cardiopulmonary resuscitation (CPR) incorrectly

Answers can be found in Appendix F.

Skill Application 11–5 Getting to Know Your Profession

Research two health care professions that interest you. Look on the Internet for their national or local offices and obtain their scope of practice and code of ethics. In addition, obtain the information needed to contact the malpractice insurance carrier for that profession. (You will need this for the next activity.)

Scope of practice: _____

_____

_____

Code of ethics: _____

_____

_____

Skill Application 11–6 Malpractice Insurance

Contact the insurance carrier from the information you received in the previous activity and request a student malpractice policy and application be sent to you. Highlight the important points and coverage of that policy below and share with your class.

_____

_____

_____

_____

_____

The Patient Care Partnership

When a patient requires health care, the quality of that care is enhanced with a true partnership between the patient and the health care institution. The American Hospital Association has developed the Patient Care Partnership document (replacing AHA's Patients' Bill of Rights), which assists all parties (patient, family members, and the health care institution) in defining and understanding their expectations, rights, and responsibilities. This document is available on AHA's website at http://www.aha.org.

Patients and their family members should be aware of their basic rights, often referred to as the Patient Care Partnership.

A brief summary of these basic rights include the right to the following:

- Considerate and respectful care
- Be told about the care that they will receive
- Examine the costs of their care
- Have their privacy protected
- Be involved in decisions concerning their care
- Be able to accept or refuse any treatment or procedure
- Be told of hospital rules and regulations

Although many may think of health care as confined to the hospital, this is far from accurate. With the many recent changes in health care in the United States, more and more care is occurring in outpatient clinics, rehabilitation centers, physicians' offices, and long-term care facilities. Long-term care facility residents have an additional set of rights that are guaranteed to them. These rights are listed in a document called the Resident's Bill of Rights and include the following:

- Residents can freely choose their physician, treatment, and care, and decide whether they will participate in any research project.
- Residents are protected from any type of abuse or chemical and physical restraints. Chemical restraints include sedatives to "control" the patient and make it easier to care for them.
- Residents should have a choice in their activities and schedules.
- Residents can voice criticism or complaints without any fear of retaliation.
- Residents can organize in groups for purposes of religious or social activities.
- Residents have access to information on their medical benefits and records. In addition, they can look at evaluation results of the long-term facility, including any identified deficiencies.
- Residents can manage their own moneys and possessions.
- Residents have unlimited access to their immediate family and relatives. If a married couple is staying at the facility, they have the right to share a room.

Understanding Patient's Wishes

An important part of the patient care partnership is clear communication of their health care wishes. Modern medicine may have the ability to prolong a life with advanced technology, but some patients choose to die naturally. Patients with no hope of recovery can request that no extra measures be given to resuscitate them.

Patients may have an **advance directive** signed. This is often called a **living will** because it states the patient's wishes concerning the handling of their body while still living. For example, it specifies what can and cannot be done to sustain life if the patient cannot make that decision. This can occur with a patient who is unconscious and in a vegetative state or someone who has just stopped breathing. Figure 11–6 is an example of health care directive.

Patients can also give others the ability to make decisions for them if they are unable to. This is a called a **health care proxy**, which is a legal document that identifies someone else to make the decisions for them. A legal document that identifies another individual to make decisions for the patient if they are unable to is called **durable power of attorney**. Figure 11–7 is an example of a durable power of attorney for health care.

Living wills often result in a notation in the chart or a physician order specifying the patient's wishes. For example, the physician may write an order in the chart that states "do not resuscitate" (DNR).

Health Care Directive

Directive made this _____ day of _____ , _____ .
(Year)

I, _____ being of sound mind, willfully, and voluntarily make known my desire that my dying

shall not be artificially prolonged under the circumstances set forth below, and do hereby declare that:

(A) If at any time I should have an incurable and irreversible condition certified to be a terminal condition by my attending physician, and where the application of life-sustaining treatment would serve only to artificially prolong the process of my dying, I direct that such treatment be withheld or withdrawn, and that I be permitted to die naturally. I understand "terminal condition" means an incurable and irreversible condition caused by injury, disease or illness that would, within reasonable medical judgment, cause death within a reasonable period of time in accordance with accepted medical standards.

(B) If I should be in an irreversible coma or persistent vegetative state, or other permanent unconscious condition as certified by two physicians, and from which those physicians believe that I have no reasonable probability of recovery, I direct that life-sustaining treatment be withheld or withdrawn.

(C) If I am diagnosed to be in a terminal or permanent unconscious condition, [*Choose one*]

I want _____ do not want _____
artificially administered nutrition and hydration to be withdrawn or withheld the same as other forms of life-sustaining treatment. I understand artificially administered nutrition and hydration is a form of life-sustaining treatment in certain circumstances. I request all health care providers who care for me to honor this directive.

(D) In the absence of my ability to give directions regarding the use of such life-sustaining procedures, it is my intention that this directive shall be honored by my family, physicians and other health care providers as the final expression of my fundamental right to refuse medical or surgical treatment, and also honored by any person appointed to make these decisions for me, whether by durable power of attorney or otherwise. I accept the consequences of such refusal.

(E) If I have been diagnosed as pregnant and that diagnosis is known to my physician, this directive shall have no force or effect during the course of my pregnancy.

(F) I understand the full import of this directive and I am emotionally and mentally competent to make this directive. I also understand that I may amend or revoke this directive at any time.

(G) I make the following additional directions regarding my care:

_____

_____

_____

_____

Signed: _____

The declarer has been personally known to me and I believe him or her to be of sound mind. In addition, I am not the attending physician, an employee of the attending physician or health care facility in which the declarer is a patient, or any person who has a claim against any portion of the estate of the declarer upon the declarer's decease at the time of the execution of the directive.

Witness: _____

Witness: _____

Figure 11–6
Sample health care directive.

Durable Power of Attorney for Health Care

Notice to Person Executing This Document

This is an important legal document. Before executing this document you should know these facts:

- This document gives the person you designate as your Health Care Agent the power to make MOST <u>health</u> care decisions for you if you lose the capability to make informed health care decisions for yourself. This power is effective only when you lose the capacity to make informed health care decisions for yourself. As long as you have the capacity to make informed health care decisions for yourself, you retain the right to make all medical and other health care decisions.

- You may include specific limitations in this document on the authority of the Health Care Agent to make health care decisions for you.

- Subject to any specific limitations you include in this document, if you do lose the capacity to make an informed decision on a health care matter, the Health Care Agent *GENERALLY* will be authorized by this document to make health care decisions for you to the same extent as you could make those decisions yourself, if you had the capacity to do so. The authority of the Health Care Agent to make health care decisions for you *GENERALLY* will include the authority to give informed consent, to refuse to give informed consent, or to withdraw informed consent to any care, treatment, service, or procedure to maintain, diagnose, or treat a physical or mental condition. You can limit that right in this document if you choose.

- A Health Care Agent can only act under state law. "Mercy killing" is not allowed under Washington state law. A Health Care Agent will **NEVER** be allowed to authorize "mercy killing," euthanasia or any procedure which would actually speed up the natural process of dying.

- When exercising his or her authority to make health care decisions for you when deciding on your behalf, the Health Care Agent will have to act consistent with your wishes, or if they are unknown, in your best interest. You may make your wishes known to the Health Care Agent by including them in this document or by making them known in another manner.

- When acting under this document the Health Care Agent *GENERALLY* will have the same rights that you have to receive information about proposed health care, to review health care records, and to consent to the disclosure of health care records.

1. Creation of Durable Power of Attorney for Health Care

I intend to create a power of attorney (Health Care Agent) by appointing the person or persons designated herein to make health care decisions for me to the same extent that I could make such decisions for myself if I was capable of doing so, as recognized by RCW 11.94.010. This designation becomes effective when I cannot make health care decisions for myself as determined by my attending physician or designee, such as if I am unconscious, or if I am otherwise temporarily or permanently incapable of making health care decisions. The Health Care Agent's power shall cease if and when I regain my capacity to make health care decisions.

2. Designation of Health Care Agent and Alternate Agents

If my attending physician or his or her designee determines that I am not capable of giving informed consent to health care, I _____, designate and appoint:

Name_____ Address _____

City_____ State _____ Zip _____ Phone _____

as my attorney-in-fact (Health Care Agent) by granting him or her the Durable Power of Attorney for Health Care recognized in RCW 11.94.010 and authorize her or him to consult with my physicians about the possibility of my regaining the capacity to make treatment decisions and to accept, plan, stop, and refuse treatment on my behalf with the treating physicians and health personnel.

In the event that _____ is unable or unwilling to serve, I grant these powers to

Name_____ Address _____

City_____ State _____ Zip _____ Phone _____

In the event that both _____ and _____

are unable or unwilling to serve, I grant these powers to

Name_____ Address _____

City_____ State _____ Zip _____ Phone _____

Figure 11–7

Sample durable power of attorney for health care.

Your name (print)_____

3. General Statement of Authority Granted.

My Health Care Agent is specifically authorized to give informed consent for health care treatment when I am not capable of doing so. This includes but is not limited to consent to initiate, continue, discontinue, or forgo medical care and treatment including artificially supplied nutrition and hydration, following and interpreting my instructions for the provision, withholding, or withdrawing of life-sustaining treatment, which are contained in any Health Care Directive or other form of "living will" I may have executed or elsewhere, and to receive and consent to the release of medical information. When the Health Care Agent does not have any stated desires or instructions from me to follow, he or she shall act in my best interest in making health care decisions.

The above authorization to make health care decisions does not include the following absent a court order:

(1) Therapy or other procedure given for the purpose of inducing convulsion;

(2) Surgery solely for the purpose of psychosurgery;

(3) Commitment to or placement in a treatment facility for the mentally ill, except pursuant to the provisions of Chapter 71.05 RCW;

(4) Sterilization.

I hereby revoke any prior grants of durable power of attorney for health care.

4. Special Provisions

_____

_____

_____

_____

_____

DATED this _____ day of _____ , _____ .
(Year)

GRANTOR _____

STATE OF WASHINGTON   )
)ss.
(COUNTY OF _____)

I certify that I know or have satisfactory evidence that the GRANTOR, _____

signed this instrument and acknowledged it to be his or her free and voluntary act for the uses and purposes mentioned in the instrument.

DATED this _____ day of _____ , _____ .
(Year)

_____
NOTARY PUBLIC in and for the State of Washington,

residing at _____

My commission expires _____

Figure 11–7
(Continued)

It is important to know whether your patient has this order in the event that they cease to breathe or the heart stops during your treatment or interaction.

Insuring Competent Care

Insuring that all health care at a health care facility is given by competent individuals is a critical part of the health care partnership to develop patient confidence. Most health care professionals are licensed, meaning they have met the requirements set forth by their governing body. Some professionals must obtain a degree through an accredited college and others require the degree plus completion of an exam. It is important that you are aware of the requirements for your profession in your particular state, as some requirements vary from state to state. Your professional organization is a great place to start inquiring about these requirements. Maintaining your license may be a matter of renewing and paying a fee or perhaps a certain number of **continuing education** credits are required in a certain time period. It is important to keep those licenses current. Continuing education are classes, webinars, journal articles with exams, in-services, or any other educational program that you complete. These activities keep you current and up-to-date in your practice. Think about it, would you want to be cared for by someone who graduated in 1974 and never attended another educational activity? Probably not. Health care changes and advances daily and you must stay current in order to provide the best care to your patients.

Certification is often achieved by obtaining training or education beyond or in addition to your initial degree; some examples include CPR, advanced cardiac life support (ACLS), or pediatric advanced life support (PALS) to just name a few. You should be aware of the certifications that are required for your position and maintain them, meaning do not let them expire! It is your responsibility to keep all licenses and certification current. It is part of your professional responsibility to your employer and your patients to remain current in your license and certification.

Some Final Thoughts as You Complete This Text

Throughout this worktext we discussed how to showcase or "brand" yourself. Now that you have obtained employment, it is more important than ever to showcase yourself as someone with a positive, trustworthy attitude who places customer service (patient care) first. All of the items we discussed regarding being on time, having a neat and tidy appearance, and a pleasant demeanor, to name a few, continue to be important. Most people change careers or jobs three or four times in their life; you never know who is watching you, who

Skill Application 11–7 **Certification**

List three certifications that you wish to obtain after graduation. Find the website for these three certifications, write them down along with the requirements for each.

1. Certification:_____

 Website: _____

 Requirements: _____

2. Certification:_____

 Website: _____

 Requirements: _____

3. Certification:_____

 Website: _____

 Requirements: _____

will notice you, or where you will go next. Being a professional in each interaction will ensure your continued success as you climb the career ladder.

Customer service is an important part of being a professional; our patients are consumers of health care. Your patients come from many different backgrounds with many different experiences and talents. Not all patients will be your favorites, but all patients deserve your respect. You should consider caring for patients an honor and privilege and strive to provide the best care possible. A few tips include the following:

- Call your patient by their proper name on the medical record until they direct you otherwise.
- Always provide privacy, pull the curtain, or close the door.
- Be compassionate, empathetic, and kind.
- Introduce yourself and explain any procedure prior to implementing it.
- Ask permission before touching a patient.
- Strive to always use common sense and common courtesy.

By implementing these few small things, you can make a positive impression on the patient, your customer.

Summary

Obtaining your first professional position means the work continues. There are issues that many health professions have in common.

- Medical ethics must be considered by all current and future health care professionals.

- Confidentiality, respect, and trust coupled with safe and appropriate care will serve as guidelines for ethical treatment of patients.

- Your patients will be faced with issues such as death and dying, euthanasia, and other issues that will cause examination of your personal beliefs.

- Legal issues are also an important consideration for all health care practitioners. It is important to understand your particular scope of practice so that you understand what it is you can and cannot do. You must also understand the terms *negligence* and *malpractice* and prevent their occurrences in the practice of your chosen profession.

A summary of standards that will protect you and the patient follows:

1. Know your scope of practice and keep within it.

2. Remain current with your knowledge and use only approved, correct procedures.

3. Know and follow your institution's policies and procedures concerning informed consent.

4. Know your institution's safety policies and procedures. Especially important are fire safety, patient transportation, and handling of accidents, hazardous materials, and defective equipment.

5. Keep all information confidential and give considerate care to all patients.

6. Maintain a professional image in dress and attitude.

7. Report any errors or accidents immediately, and document them with an incident report.

8. Do not accept money or tips for any services.

9. Remain current in your licensing, certification, and continuing education mandates.

10. Continue to showcase yourself in a positive light.

11. Customer service should be considered with each patient encounter. Remember it is a privilege to provide patient care.

Case Study | **11–1**

You are working in an outpatient surgery clinic. In the hallway you hear two of your coworkers discussing the cosmetic surgery that one of the patients is receiving. This is not a medical discussion and is more of a gossip session with derogatory comments concerning the patient's vanity. They are speaking loudly enough that you feel people in the visitors' waiting area can hear their conversation. What should you do in this situation?

_____

_____

_____

Case Study 11–2

During the COVID-19 pandemic, it was determined that COVID-19 was transmitted by close contact and airborne transmission. Discuss some of the infection control practices that Americans were encouraged to use to prevent the spread of COVID-19.

_____

_____

_____

_____

Internet Activity

Using Internet search engines, find additional material on selected topics that can help you and your fellow students. Some suggested keywords are medical ethics, HIPAA regulations, euthanasia, malpractice, and hospice. Write down something new that you found to share.

_____

_____

_____

_____

Appendix A

Health Care Websites

Government Resources

Americans with Disabilities

www.ada.gov
This government website provides helpful information regarding the Americans with Disabilities Act. It contains videos and publications that help explain the law.

Centers for Disease Control and Prevention (CDC)

http://www.cdc.gov
This is a government website that contains information and statistics on diseases, prevention, and public health. The CDC detects and responds to new and emerging health threats, tackling the biggest health problems causing death and disability for Americans. It also promotes healthy and safe behaviors, communities, and environments.

Centers for Medicare and Medicaid Services

www.cms.gov
This is the government website that provides information regarding Medicare and Medicaid. It contains helpful links regarding education and research along with providing enrollment options for those needing health care insurance.

Food and Drug Administration

http://www.fda.gov
This site has information on topics such as specific drugs, recalls and product safety, and postmarket drug safety.

Health Insurance Marketplace

https://www.healthcare.gov
This is a federal government website that provides consumers and providers with information regarding the Affordable Care Act.

Occupational Safety and Health Administration

https://www.osha.gov
United States Department of Labor, Occupational Safety and Health Administration. This is a government website that contains a description of OSHA, its services, and documents pertaining to worker's rights. This site is of particular interest to health care workers due to the content on blood-borne pathogen exposure, prevention, and treatment.

National Institutes of Health

http://www.nih.gov
National Institutes of Health (NIH) is a branch of the United States Department of Health and Human Services. The mission of the NIH is to seek fundamental knowledge about the nature and behavior of living systems and the application of knowledge to enhance health, lengthen life, and reduce illness and disability.

Health Care Regulating Bodies

The Agency for Healthcare Research and Quality

http://www.ahrq.gov
The Agency for Healthcare Research and Quality is a service of the United States Department of Health and Human Services. On this site, you can choose the "For Professionals" link and find tools, recommendations, and resources to help guide practice.

CARF International

https://www.carf.org/home/
Provide accreditation for rehabilitation for a disability, treatment for addiction and substance abuse, home and community services, retirement living, or other health and human services.

The Joint Commission

http://www.jointcommission.org
The Joint Commission is an independent, not-for-profit organization that accredits and certifies more than 20,500 health care organizations and programs in the United States. On this website, you can find information on accreditation standards, education on topics such as hospital-acquired infections, and also you can find accredited organizations or make complaints about organizations.

Educational Resources

Harvard Health

www.health.harvard.edu
This education website allows you to sign up for e-mail newsletters. This site contains links and information on many health conditions. Content is reviewed and approved by Harvard health experts.

Medline

http://www.medlineplus.gov
This government website assists consumers in locating health information.

Physician Desk Reference

http://www.pdrhealth.com
This site for consumers from the PDR includes information about prescription and nonprescription drugs, herbal medicines, and supplements.

The Internet Drug Index

https://www.rxlist.com
This website is an online medical resource that offers detailed and current pharmaceutical information on brand and generic drugs.

The Mayo Clinic

http://www.mayoclinic.org
This website is maintained by the Mayo Clinic's experts and is an excellent source of health information for consumers and professionals.

UpToDate

www.uptodate.com
This website is an evidence-based clinical decision support resource designed to be used at the point of care. Some content requires a subscription.

Professional Organizations

American Association of Medical Assistants

http://www.aama-ntl.org
The website is for medical assisting professionals.

American Association of Pharmacy Technicians

http://www.pharmacytechnician.com
The professional association for pharmacy technicians. This site contains a helpful career center.

American Association of Professional Coders

www.aapc.com
The largest training and credentialing organization for the business side of health care.

American Association for Respiratory Care

www.aarc.org
The professional organization that represents respiratory therapists.

American Dental Hygienist Association

http://www.adha.org
The dental hygienist professional organization, which includes options for students and promotes oral health.

American Massage Therapy Association

http://www.amtamassage.org
A professional organization for massage therapist, which includes educational links and scholarship information.

American Nurses Associations

www.nursingworld.org
A professional organization for registered nurses. This site contains many educational links, a career section, and a large section on health care ethics.

Association of Surgical Technologists

http://www.ast.org
The professional organization for surgical technologists provides education, a career center, and information on public health policy.

Medical Technology Programs

https://www.medicaltechnologyschools.com/
This website allows you to search for many medical technology programs and careers.

Nursing Assistant Resources on the Web

http://www.nursingassistants.net
This website is a repository for helpful links, educational articles, and advice for CNAs.

National Association of Health Care Assistants

http://nahcacareforce.org
The professional organization of and for CNAs.

National Federation of Licensed Practical Nurses

http://www.nflpn.org
The professional organization for licensed practical nurses and licensed vocational nurses. This site includes membership options for students.

Radiology.org

http://www.radiology.org/associations
This site provides a comprehensive listing of and links to radiology associations and societies. It also lists radiology journals and companies with links to the website of each.

Society of Medical Diagnostic Sonography

http://www.sdms.org
Professional organization for ultrasound professionals.

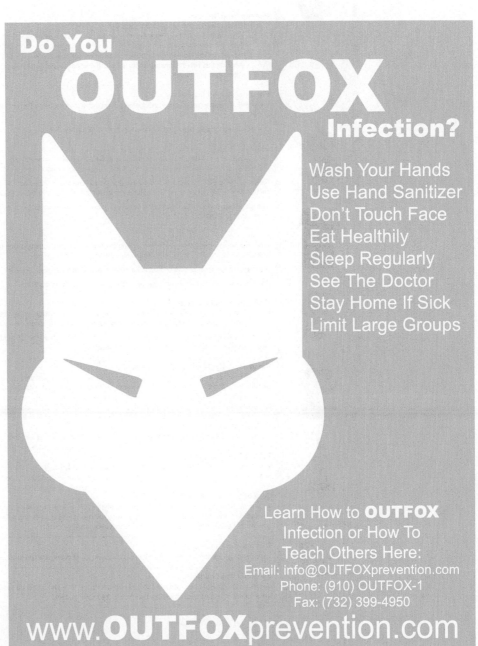

Figure B-1
CDC's OUTFOX prevention campaign poster.

STANDARD PRECAUTIONS

Assume that every person is potentially infected or colonized with an organism that could be transmitted in the healthcare setting and apply the following infection control practices.

ATTENTION!

Hand Hygiene

Avoid unnecessary touching of surfaces in close proximity to the patient.

When hands are visibly dirty, contaminated with proteinaceous material, or visibly soiled with blood or body fluids, wash hands with soap and water.

If hands are not visibly soiled, or after removing visible material with soap and water, decontaminate hands with alcohol-based hand rub. Alternatively, hands may be washed with an antimicrobial soap and water.

Perform Hand Hygiene:
- Before having direct contact with patients
- After contact with blood, body fluids, or excretions, mucous membranes, non-intact skin, or wound dressings
- After contact with a patient's intact skin (e.g. when taking a pulse or blood pressure or lifting a patient)
- If hands will be moving from a contaminated body site to a clean body site during patient care
- After contact with inanimate objects (including medical equipment) in the immediate vicinity of the patient
- After removing gloves

Personal Protect Equipment (PPE)

Wear PPE when the nature of the anticipated patient interaction indicates that contact with blood or body fluids may occur.

Before leaving the patient's room or cubicle, remove and discard PPE.

Gloves

Wear gloves when contact with blood or other potentially infectious materials, mucous membranes, non-intact skin, or potentially contaminated intact skin (e.g. of a patient incontinent of stool or urine) could occur.

Remove gloves after contact with a patient and/or the surrounding environment using proper technique to prevent hand contamination. Do not wear the same pair of gloves for the care of more than one patient.

Change gloves during patient care if the hands will move from a contaminated body site (e.g. perineal area) to a clean body site (e.g. face).

Gowns

Wear a gown to protect skin and prevent soiling or contamination of clothing during procedures and patient-care activities when contact with blood, body fluids, secretions, or excretions is anticipated.

Wear a gown for direct patient contact if the patient has uncontained secretions or excretions.

Remove gown and perform hand hygiene before leaving patient's environment.

Mouth, Nose, Eye Protection

Use PPE to protect the mucous membranes of the eyes, nose and mouth during procedures and patient-care activities that are likely to generate splashes or sprays of blood, body fluids, secretions or excretions.

During aerosol-generating procedures wear one of the following: a face shield that fully covers the front and sides of the face, a mask with attached shield, or a mask and goggles.

Respiratory Hygiene/Cough Etiquette

Educate healthcare personnel to contain respiratory secretions to prevent droplet and fomite transmission of respiratory pathogens, especially during seasonal outbreaks of viral respiratory tract infections.
Offer masks to coughing patients and other symptomatic persons (e.g. persons who accompany ill patients) upon entry into the facility.

Patient Placement

Include the potential for transmission of infectious agents in patient-placement decisions.

Patient-Care Equipment and Instruments/Devices

Wear PPE (e.g. gloves, gown) according to the level of anticipated contamination, when handling patient-care equipment and instruments/devices that are visibly soiled or may have been in contact with blood or body fluids.

Care of the Environment

Include multi-use electronic equipment in policies and procedures for preventing contamination and for cleaning and disinfection, especially those items that are used by patients, those used during delivery of patient care, and mobile devices that are moved in and out of patient rooms frequently (e.g. daily).

Textiles and Laundry

Hand used textiles and fabrics with minimum agitation to avoid contamination of air, surfaces and persons.

Safe injection practices

Needles, cannulae and syringes are sterile, single-use items; they should not be reused for another patient nor to access a medication or solution that might be used for a subsequent patient.

Source: CDC/Centers for Disease Control and Prevention.

Figure B-2
Standard precautions.

GUIDELINE FOR ISOLATION PRECAUTIONS (2007): Preventing Transmission of Infectious Agents in Healthcare Settings

Standard Precautions

IV. Standard Precautions
Assume that every person is potentially infected or colonized with an organism that could be transmitted in the healthcare setting and apply the following infection control practices during the delivery of health care.

IV.A. Hand Hygiene
IV.A.1. During the delivery of healthcare, avoid unnecessary touching of surfaces in close proximity to the patient to prevent both contamination of clean hands from environmental surfaces and transmission of pathogens from contaminated hands to surfaces.
IV.A.2. When hands are visibly dirty, contaminated with proteinaceous material, or visibly soiled with blood or body fluids, wash hands with either a nonantimicrobial soap and water or an antimicrobial soap and water.
IV.A.3. If hands are not visibly soiled, or after removing visible material with nonantimicrobial soap and water, decontaminate hands in the clinical situations described in IV.A.2.a-f. The preferred method of hand decontamination is with an alcohol-based hand rub. Alternatively, hands may be washed with an antimicrobial soap and water. Frequent use of alcohol-based hand rub immediately following handwashing with nonantimicrobial soap may increase the frequency of dermatitis.
IV.A.3.a. Before having direct contact with patients.
IV.A.3.b. After contact with blood, body fluids or excretions, mucous membranes, nonintact skin, or wound dressings.
IV.A.3.c. After contact with a patient's intact skin (e.g., when taking a pulse or blood pressure or lifting a patient).
IV.A.3.d. If hands will be moving from a contaminated-body site to a clean-body site during patient care.
IV.A.3.e. After contact with inanimate objects (including medical equipment) in the immediate vicinity of the patient.
IV.A.3.f. After removing gloves.
IV.A.4. Wash hands with non-antimicrobial soap and water or with antimicrobial soap and water if contact with spores (e.g., *C. difficile* or *Bacillus anthracis*) is likely to have occurred. The physical action of washing and rinsing hands under such circumstances is recommended because alcohols, chlorhexidine, iodophors, and other antiseptic agents have poor activity against spores.
IV.A.5. Do not wear artificial fingernails or extenders if duties include direct contact with patients at high risk for infection and associated adverse outcomes (e.g., those in ICUs or operating rooms).
IV.A.5.a. Develop an organizational policy on the wearing of non-natural nails by healthcare personnel who have direct contact with patients outside of the groups specified above.

IV.B. Personal protective equipment (PPE)
IV.B.1. Observe the following principles of use:
IV.B.1.a. Wear PPE, as described in IV.B.2-4, when the nature of the anticipated patient interaction indicates that contact with blood or body fluids may occur.
IV.B.1.b. Prevent contamination of clothing and skin during the process of removing PPE (see Figure).
IV.B.1.c. Before leaving the patient's room or cubicle, remove and discard PPE.
IV.B.2. Gloves
IV.B.2.a. Wear gloves when it can be reasonably anticipated that contact with blood or other potentially infectious materials, mucous membranes, nonintact skin, or potentially contaminated intact skin (e.g., of a patient incontinent of stool or urine) could occur.
IV.B.2.b. Wear gloves with fit and durability appropriate to the task.
IV.B.2.b.i. Wear disposable medical examination gloves for providing direct patient care.
IV.B.2.b.ii. Wear disposable medical examination gloves or reusable utility gloves for cleaning the environment or medical equipment.
IV.B.2.c. Remove gloves after contact with a patient and/or the surrounding environment (including medical equipment) using proper technique to prevent hand contamination. Do not wear the same pair of gloves for the care of more than one patient. Do not wash gloves for the purpose of reuse since this practice has been associated with transmission of pathogens.
IV.B.2.d. Change gloves during patient care if the hands will move from a contaminated body-site (e.g., perineal area) to a clean body-site (e.g., face).
IV.B.3. Gowns
IV.B.3.a. Wear a gown, that is appropriate to the task, to protect skin and prevent soiling or contamination of clothing during procedures and patient-care activities when contact with blood, body fluids, secretions, or excretions is anticipated.
IV.B.3.a.i. Wear a gown for direct patient contact if the patient has uncontained secretions or excretions.
IV.B.3.a.ii. Remove gown and perform hand hygiene before leaving the patient's environment.
IV.B.3.b. Do not reuse gowns, even for repeated contacts with the same patient.
IV.B.3.c. Routine donning of gowns upon entrance into a high risk unit (e.g., ICU, NICU, HSCT unit) is not indicated.
IV.B.4. Mouth, nose, eye protection
IV.B.4.a. Use PPE to protect the mucous membranes of the eyes, nose and mouth during procedures and patient-care activities that are likely to generate splashes or sprays of blood, body fluids, secretions and excretions. Select masks, goggles, face shields, and combinations of each according to the need anticipated by the task performed.
IV.B.5. During aerosol-generating procedures (e.g., bronchoscopy, suctioning of the respiratory tract [if not using in-line suction catheters], endotracheal intubation) in patients who are not suspected of being infected with an agent for which respiratory protection is otherwise recommended (e.g., *M. tuberculosis*, SARS or hemorrhagic fever viruses), wear one of the following: a face shield that fully covers the front and sides of the face, a mask with attached shield, or a mask and goggles (in addition to gloves and gown).

IV.C. Respiratory Hygiene/Cough Etiquette
IV.C.1. Educate healthcare personnel on the importance of source control measures to contain respiratory secretions to prevent droplet and fomite transmission of respiratory pathogens, especially during seasonal outbreaks of viral respiratory tract infections (e.g., influenza, RSV, adenovirus, parainfluenza virus) in communities.
IV.C.2. Implement the following measures to contain respiratory secretions in patients and accompanying individuals who have signs and symptoms of a respiratory infection, beginning at the point of initial encounter in a healthcare setting (e.g., triage, reception and waiting areas in emergency departments, outpatient clinics and physician offices.
IV.C.2.a. Post signs at entrances and in strategic places (e.g., elevators, cafeterias) within ambulatory and inpatient settings with instructions to patients and other persons with symptoms of a respiratory infection to cover their mouths/noses when coughing or sneezing, use and dispose of tissues, and perform hand hygiene after hands have been in contact with respiratory secretions.
IV.C.2.b. Provide tissues and no-touch receptacles (e.g., foot-pedal-operated lid or open, plastic-lined waste basket) for disposal of tissues.

Compiled by OUTFOX Prevention
OPSP1 ©2012 OUTFOX Prevention

IV.C.2.c. Provide resources and instructions for performing hand hygiene in or near waiting areas in ambulatory and inpatient settings; provide conveniently-located dispensers of alcohol-based hand rubs and, where sinks are available, supplies for handwashing.
IV.C.2.d. During periods of increased prevalence of respiratory infections in the community (e.g., as indicated by increased school absenteeism, increased number of patients seeking care for a respiratory infection), offer masks to coughing patients and other symptomatic persons (e.g., persons who accompany ill patients) upon entry into the facility or medical office and encourage them to maintain special separation, ideally a distance of at least 3 feet, from others in common waiting areas.
IV.C.2.d.i. Some facilities may find it logistically easier to institute this recommendation year-round as a standard of practice.

IV.D. Patient placement
IV.D.1. Include the potential for transmission of infectious agents in patient-placement decisions. Place patients who pose a risk for transmission to others (e.g., uncontained secretions, excretions or wound drainage; infants with suspected viral respiratory or gastrointestinal infections) in a single-patient room when available.
IV.D.2. Determine patient placement based on the following principles:
-Route(s) of transmission of the known or suspected infectious agent
-Risk factors for transmission in the infected patient
-Risk factors for adverse outcomes resulting from an HAI in other patients in the area or room being considered for patient-placement
-Availability of single-patient rooms
-Patient options for room-sharing (e.g., cohorting patients with the same infection)

IV.E. Patient-care equipment and instruments/devices
IV.E.1. Establish policies and procedures for containing, transporting, and handling patient-care equipment and instruments/devices that may be contaminated with blood or body fluids.
IV.E.2. Remove organic material from critical and semi-critical instrument/devices, using recommended cleaning agents before high level disinfection and sterilization to enable effective disinfection and sterilization processes.
IV.E.3. Wear PPE (e.g., gloves, gown), according to the level of anticipated contamination, when handling patient-care equipment and instruments/devices that is visibly soiled or may have been in contact with blood or body fluids.

IV.F. Care of the environment
IV.F.1. Establish policies and procedures for routine and targeted cleaning of environmental surfaces as indicated by the level of patient contact and degree of soiling.
IV.F.2. Clean and disinfect surfaces that are likely to be contaminated with pathogens, including those that are in close proximity to the patient (e.g., bed rails, over bed tables) and frequently-touched surfaces in the patient care environment (e.g., door knobs, surfaces in and surrounding toilets in patients' rooms) on a more frequent schedule compared to that for other surfaces (e.g., horizontal surfaces in waiting rooms).
IV.F.3. Use EPA-registered disinfectants that have microbiocidal (i.e., killing) activity against the pathogens most likely to contaminate the patient-care environment. Use in accordance with manufacturer's instructions.
IV.F.3.a. Review the efficacy of in-use disinfectants when evidence of continuing transmission of an infectious agent (e.g., rotavirus, *C. difficile*, norovirus) may indicate resistance to the in-use product and change to a more effective disinfectant as indicated.
IV.F.4. In facilities that provide health care to pediatric patients or have waiting areas with child play toys (e.g., obstetric/gynecology offices and clinics), establish policies and procedures for cleaning and disinfecting toys at regular intervals.
Use the following principles in developing this policy and procedures:
-Select play toys that can be easily cleaned and disinfected
 -Do not permit use of stuffed furry toys if they will be shared
 -Clean and disinfect large stationary toys (e.g., climbing equipment) at least weekly and whenever visibly soiled
 -If toys are likely to be mouthed, rinse with water after disinfection; alternatively wash in a dishwasher
 -When a toy requires cleaning and disinfection, do so immediately or store in a designated labeled container separate from toys that are clean and ready for use
IV.F.5. Include multi-use electronic equipment in policies and procedures for preventing contamination and for cleaning and disinfection, especially those items that are used by patients, those used during delivery of patient care, and mobile devices that are moved in and out of patient rooms frequently (e.g., daily).
IV.F.5.a. No recommendation for use of removable protective covers or washable keyboards. *Unresolved issue*

IV.G. Textiles and laundry
IV.G.1. Handle used textiles and fabrics with minimum agitation to avoid contamination of air, surfaces and persons.
IV.G.2. If laundry chutes are used, ensure that they are properly designed, maintained, and used in a manner to minimize dispersion of aerosols from contaminated laundry.

IV.H. Safe injection practices
The following recommendations apply to the use of needles, cannulas that replace needles, and, where applicable intravenous delivery systems
IV.H.1. Use aseptic technique to avoid contamination of sterile injection equipment.
IV.H.2. Do not administer medications from a syringe to multiple patients, even if the needle or cannula on the syringe is changed. Needles, cannulae and syringes are sterile, single-use items; they should not be reused for another patient nor to access a medication or solution that might be used for a subsequent patient.
IV.H.3. Use fluid infusion and administration sets (i.e., intravenous bags, tubing and connectors) for one patient only and dispose appropriately after use. Consider a syringe or needle/cannula contaminated once it has been used to enter or connect to a patient's intravenous infusion bag or administration set.
IV.H.4. Use single-dose vials for parenteral medications whenever possible .
IV.H.5. Do not administer medications from single-dose vials or ampules to multiple patients or combine leftover contents for later use.
IV.H.6. If multidose vials must be used, both the needle or cannula and syringe used to access the multidose vial must be sterile.
IV.H.7. Do not keep multidose vials in the immediate patient treatment area and store in accordance with the manufacturer's recommendations; discard if sterility is compromised or questionable.
IV.H.8. Do not use bags or bottles of intravenous solution as a common source of supply for multiple patients.
IV.I. Infection control practices for special lumbar puncture procedures
Wear a surgical mask when placing a catheter or injecting material into the spinal canal or subdural space (i.e., during myelograms, lumbar puncture and spinal or epidural anesthesia).
Worker safety
Adhere to federal and state requirements for protection of healthcare personnel from exposure to bloodborne pathogens.

Compiled by OUTFOX Prevention
OPSP1 ©2012 OUTFOX Prevention

Figure B-2
(continued)

AIRBORNE PRECAUTIONS

(Airborne Precautions are in addition to Standard Precautions. See Standard Precautions for questions)

ATTENTION!

ATTENTION! VISITORS must report to the nurse station before entering.

Patient Placement
Private room, if possible. Ensure that patients are physically separated (i.e., >3 feet apart) from each other. Draw the privacy curtain between beds to minimize opportunities for direct contact.

Personal Protective Equipment (PPE)
Don gown upon entry into the room or cubicle. Remove gown and observe hand hygiene before leaving the patient-care environment.

Hand Hygiene (according to Standard Precautions)
Avoid unnecessary touching of surfaces in close proximity to the patient.

When hands are visibly dirty, contaminated with proteinaceous material, or visibly soiled with blood or body fluids, wash hands with soap and water.

If hands are not visibly soiled, or after removing visible material with soap and water, decontaminate hands with alcohol-based hand rub. Alternatively, hands may be washed with an antimicrobial soap and water.

Perform Hand Hygiene:
  -Before having direct contact with patients
  -After contact with blood, body fluids, or excretions, mucous membranes, non-intact skin, or wound dressings
  -After contact with a patient's intact skin (e.g. when taking a pulse or blood pressure or lifting a patient)
  -If hands will be moving from a contaminated body site to a clean body site during patient care
  -After contact with inanimate objects (including medical equipment) in the immediate vicinity of the patient
  -After removing gloves

Patient Transport
Limit transport and movement of patients outside of the room to medically-necessary purposes.

When transport or movement in any healthcare setting is necessary, ensure that infected or colonized areas of the patient's body are contained and covered.

Remove and dispose of contaminated PPE and perform hand hygiene before and after transporting patients on Contact Precautions.

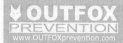
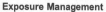

Exposure Management
Immunize or provide the appropriate immune globulin to susceptible persons as soon as possible following unprotected contact (i.e., exposed) to a patient with specific conditions (see full description).

OUTFOX PREVENTION
www.OUTFOXprevention.com

OPCP1 ©2012 OUTFOX Prevention

Source: CDC/Centers for Disease Control and Prevention.

Figure B-3
Airborne precautions.

AIRBORNE PRECAUTIONS
From: 2007 Guideline for Isolation Precautions: Preventing Transmission of Infectious Agents in Healthcare Settings

V.D. Airborne Precautions

V.D.1. Use Airborne Precautions as recommended in Appendix A for patients known or suspected to be infected with infectious agents transmitted person-to-person by the airborne route (e.g., M tuberculosis, measles, chickenpox, disseminated herpes zoster.

V.D.2. Patient placement

V.D.2.a. In *acute care hospitals and long-term care settings*, place patients who require Airborne Precautions in an AIIR that has been constructed in accordance with current guidelines.

V.D.2.a.i. Provide at least six (existing facility) or 12 (new construction/renovation) air changes per hour.

V.D.2.a.ii. Direct exhaust of air to the outside. If it is not possible to exhaust air from an AIIR directly to the outside, the air may be returned to the air-handling system or adjacent spaces if all air is directed through HEPA filters.

V.D.2.a.iii .Whenever an AIIR is in use for a patient on Airborne Precautions, monitor air pressure daily with visual indicators (e.g., smoke tubes, flutter strips), regardless of the presence of differential pressure sensing devices (e.g., manometers).

V.D.2.a.iv. Keep the AIIR door closed when not required for entry and exit.

V.D.2.b. When an AIIR is not available, transfer the patient to a facility that has an available AIIR.

V.D.2.c. In the event of an outbreak or exposure involving large numbers of patients who require Airborne Precautions:

-Consult infection control professionals before patient placement to determine the safety of alternative room that do not meet engineering requirements for an AIIR.

-Place together (cohort) patients who are presumed to have the same infection(based on clinical presentation and diagnosis when known) in areas of the facility that are away from other patients, especially patients who are at increased risk for infection (e.g., immunocompromised patients).

-Use temporary portable solutions (e.g., exhaust fan) to create a negative pressure environment in the converted area of the facility. Discharge air directly to the outside, away from people and air intakes, or direct all the air through HEPA filters before it is introduced to other air spaces.

V.D.2.d. In *ambulatory settings*:

V.D.2.d.i. Develop systems (e.g., triage, signage) to identify patients with known or suspected infections that require Airborne Precautions upon entry into ambulatory settings.

V.D.2.d.ii. Place the patient in an AIIR as soon as possible. If an AIIR is not available, place a surgical mask on the patient and place him/her in an examination room. Once the patient leaves, the room should remain vacant for the appropriate time, generally one hour, to allow for a full exchange of air.

V.D.2.d.iii. Instruct patients with a known or suspected airborne infection to wear a surgical mask and observe Respiratory Hygiene/Cough Etiquette. Once in an AIIR, the mask may be removed; the mask should remain on if the patient is not in an AIIR.

V.D.3. Personnel restrictions

Restrict susceptible healthcare personnel from entering the rooms of patients known or suspected to have measles (rubeola), varicella (chickenpox), disseminated zoster, or smallpox if other immune healthcare personnel are available.

V.D.4. Use of PPE (Personal Protective Equipment)

V.D.4.a. Wear a fit-tested NIOSH-approved N95 or higher level respirator for respiratory protection when entering the room or home of a patient when the following diseases are suspected or confirmed:

-Infectious pulmonary or laryngeal tuberculosis or when infectious tuberculosis skin lesions are present and procedures that would aerosolize viable organisms (e.g., irrigation, incision and drainage, whirlpool treatments) are performed.

-Smallpox (vaccinated and unvaccinated). Respiratory protection is recommended for all healthcare personnel, including those with a documented "take" after smallpox vaccination due to the risk of a genetically engineered virus against which the vaccine may not provide protection, or of exposure to a very large viral load (e.g., from high-risk aerosol-generating procedures, immunocompromised patients, hemorrhagic or flat smallpox).

V.D.4.b. No recommendation is made regarding the use of PPE by healthcare personnel who are presumed to be immune to measles (rubeola) or varicella-zoster based on history of disease, vaccine, or serologic testing when caring for an individual with known or suspected measles, chickenpox or disseminated zoster, due to difficulties in establishing definite immunity. Unresolved issue

V.D.4.c. No recommendation is made regarding the type of personal protective equipment (i.e., surgical mask or respiratory protection with a N95 or higher respirator) to be worn by susceptible healthcare personnel who must have contact with patients with known or suspected measles, chickenpox or disseminated herpes zoster. *Unresolved issue*

V.D.5. Patient transport

V.D.5.a. In *acute care hospitals and long-term care and other residential settings*, limit transport and movement of patients outside of the room to medically-necessary purposes.

V.D.5.b. If transport or movement outside an AIIR is necessary, instruct patients to wear a surgical mask, if possible, and observe Respiratory Hygiene/Cough Etiquette.

V.D.5.c. For patients with skin lesions associated with varicella or smallpox or draining skin lesions caused by *M. tuberculosis*, cover the affected areas to prevent aerosolization or contact with the infectious agent in skin lesions.

V.D.5.d. Healthcare personnel transporting patients who are on Airborne Precautions do not need to wear a mask or respirator during transport if the patient is wearing a mask and infectious skin lesions are covered.

V.D.6. Exposure management

Immunize or provide the appropriate immune globulin to susceptible persons as soon as possible following unprotected contact (i.e., exposed) to a patient with measles, varicella or smallpox:

-Administer measles vaccine to exposed susceptible persons within 72 hours after the exposure or administer immune globulin within six days of the exposure event for high-risk persons in whom vaccine is contraindicated.

-Administer varicella vaccine to exposed susceptible persons within 120 hours after the exposure or administer varicella immune globulin (VZIG or alternative product), when available, within 96 hours for high-risk persons in whom vaccine is contraindicated (e.g., immunocompromised patients, pregnant women, newborns whose mother's varicella onset was <5 days before or within 48 hours after delivery).

-Administer smallpox vaccine to exposed susceptible persons within 4 days after exposure.

V.D.7. Discontinue Airborne Precautions according to pathogen-specific recommendations in Appendix A.

V.D.8. Consult CDC's "Guidelines for Preventing the Transmission of *Mycobacterium tuberculosis* in Health-Care Settings, 2005" and the "Guideline for Environmental Infection Control in Health-Care Facilities" for additional guidance on environment strategies for preventing transmission of tuberculosis in healthcare settings. The environmental recommendations in these guidelines may be applied to patients with other infections that require Airborne Precautions.

OPCP1 ©2012 OUTFOX Prevention

Figure B-3
(continued)

CONTACT PRECAUTIONS

(Contact Precautions are in addition to Standard Precautions. See Standard Precautions for questions)

ATTENTION! VISITORS must report to the nurse station before entering.

Patient Placement
Private room, if possible. Ensure that patients are physically separated (i.e., >3 feet apart) from each other. Draw the privacy curtain between beds to minimize opportunities for direct contact.

Personal Protective Equipment (PPE)
Don gown upon entry into the room or cubicle. Remove gown and observe hand hygiene before leaving the patient-care environment.

Hand Hygiene (according to Standard Precautions)
Avoid unnecessary touching of surfaces in close proximity to the patient.

When hands are visibly dirty, contaminated with proteinaceous material, or visibly soiled with blood or body fluids, wash hands with soap and water.

If hands are not visibly soiled, or after removing visible material with soap and water, decontaminate hands with alcohol-based hand rub. Alternatively, hands may be washed with an antimicrobial soap and water.

Perform Hand Hygiene:
-Before having direct contact with patients
-After contact with blood, body fluids, or excretions, mucous membranes, non-intact skin, or wound dressings
-After contact with a patient's intact skin (e.g. when taking a pulse or blood pressure or lifting a patient)
-If hands will be moving from a contaminated body site to a clean body site during patient care
-After contact with inanimate objects (including medical equipment) in the immediate vicinity of the patient
-After removing gloves

Patient Transport
Limit transport and movement of patients outside of the room to medically-necessary purposes.

When transport or movement in any healthcare setting is necessary, ensure that infected or colonized areas of the patient's body are contained and covered.

Remove and dispose of contaminated PPE and perform hand hygiene before and after transporting patients on Contact Precautions.

Patient-Care Equipment and Instruments/Devices
If common use of equipment for multiple patients is unavoidable, clean and disinfect such equipment before use on another patient.

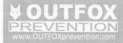

OPCP1 ©2012 OUTFOX Prevention

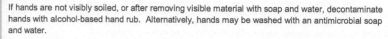

Source: CDC/Centers for Disease Control and Prevention.

Figure B-4
Contact precautions.

CONTACT PRECAUTIONS

From: 2007 Guideline for Isolation Precautions: Preventing Transmission of Infectious Agents in Healthcare Settings

V. Transmission-Based Precautions

V.B. Contact Precautions

V.B.1. Use Contact Precautions as recommended in Appendix A for patients with known or suspected infections or evidence of syndromes that represent an increased risk for contact transmission. For specific recommendations for use of Contact Precautions for colonization or infection with MDROs, go to the MDRO guideline: www.cdc.gov/ncidod/dhqp/pdf/ar/mdroGuideline2006.pdf .

V.B.2. Patient placement

V.B.2.a. In acute care hospitals, place patients who require Contact Precautions in a single-patient room when available.
When single-patient rooms are in short supply, apply the following principles for making decisions on patient placement:
-Prioritize patients with conditions that may facilitate transmission (e.g., uncontained drainage, stool incontinence) for single-patient room placement.
-Place together in the same room (cohort) patients who are infected or colonized with the same pathogen and are suitable roommates
-If it becomes necessary to place a patient who requires Contact Precautions in a room with a patient who is not infected or colonized with the same infectious agent:
-Avoid placing patients on Contact Precautions in the same room with patients who have conditions that may increase the risk of adverse outcome from infection or that may facilitate transmission (e.g., those who are immunocompromised, have open wounds, or have anticipated prolonged lengths of stay).
-Ensure that patients are physically separated (i.e., >3 feet apart) from each other. Draw the privacy curtain between beds to minimize opportunities for direct contact.)
-Change protective attire and perform hand hygiene between contact with patients in the same room, regardless of whether one or both patients are on Contact Precautions.
V.B.2.b. In long-term care and other residential settings, make decisions regarding patient placement on a case-by-case basis, balancing infection risks to other patients in the room, the presence of risk factors that increase the likelihood of transmission, and the potential adverse psychological impact on the infected or colonized patient.
V.B.2.c. In ambulatory settings, place patients who require Contact Precautions in an examination room or cubicle as soon as possible.

V.B.3. Use of personal protective equipment

V.B.3.a. Gloves Wear gloves whenever touching the patient's intact skin or surfaces and articles in close proximity to the patient (e.g., medical equipment, bed rails). Don gloves upon entry into the room or cubicle.

V.B.3.b. Gowns

V.B.3.b.i. Wear a gown whenever anticipating that clothing will have direct contact with the patient or potentially contaminated environmental surfaces or equipment in close proximity to the patient. Don gown upon entry into the room or cubicle. Remove gown and observe hand hygiene before leaving the patient-care environment.
V.B.3.b.ii. After gown removal, ensure that clothing and skin do not contact potentially contaminated environmental surfaces that could result in possible transfer of microorganism to other patients or environmental surfaces.

V.B.4. Patient transport

V.B.4.a. In acute care hospitals and long-term care and other residential settings, limit transport and movement of patients outside of the room to medically-necessary purposes.
V.B.4.b. When transport or movement in any healthcare setting is necessary, ensure that infected or colonized areas of the patient's body are contained and covered.
V.B.4.c. Remove and dispose of contaminated PPE and perform hand hygiene prior to transporting patients on Contact Precautions.
V.B.4.d. Don clean PPE to handle the patient at the transport destination.

V.B.5. Patient-care equipment and instruments/devices

V.B.5.a. Handle patient-care equipment and instruments/devices according to Standard Precautions.
V.B.5.b. In acute care hospitals and long-term care and other residential settings, use disposable noncritical patient-care equipment (e.g., blood pressure cuffs) or implement patient-dedicated use of such equipment. If common use of equipment for multiple patients is unavoidable, clean and disinfect such equipment before use on another patient.
V.B.5.c. In home care settings
V.B.5.c.i. Limit the amount of non-disposable patient-care equipment brought into the home of patients on Contact Precautions. Whenever possible, leave patient-care equipment in the home until discharge from home care services.
V.B.5.c.ii. If noncritical patient-care equipment (e.g., stethoscope) cannot remain in the home, clean and disinfect items before taking them from the home using a low- to intermediate-level disinfectant. Alternatively, place contaminated reusable items in a plastic bag for transport and subsequent cleaning and disinfection.
V.B.5.d. In ambulatory settings, place contaminated reusable noncritical patient-care equipment in a plastic bag for transport to a soiled utility area for reprocessing.

V.B.6. Environmental measures Ensure that rooms of patients on Contact Precautions are prioritized for frequent cleaning and disinfection (e.g., at least daily) with a focus on frequently-touched surfaces (e.g., bed rails, overbed table, bedside commode, lavatory surfaces in patient bathrooms, doorknobs) and equipment in the immediate vicinity of the patient.
V.B.7. Discontinue Contact Precautions after signs and symptoms of the infection have resolved or according to pathogen-specific recommendations in Appendix A.

OPCP1 ©2012 OUTFOX Prevention

Figure B-4
(continued)

DROPLET PRECAUTIONS

ATTENTION!

(Droplet Precautions are in addition to Standard Precautions. See Standard Precautions for questions)

ATTENTION! VISITORS must report to the nurse station before entering.

Patient Placement

Private room, if possible. Ensure that patients are physically separated (i.e., >3 feet apart) from each other. Draw the privacy curtain between beds to minimize opportunities for direct contact.

Personal Protective Equipment (PPE)

Don a mask upon entry into the patient room or cubicle

Hand Hygiene (according to Standard Precautions)

Avoid unnecessary touching of surfaces in close proximity to the patient.

When hands are visibly dirty, contaminated with proteinaceous material, or visibly soiled with blood or body fluids, wash hands with soap and water.

If hands are not visibly soiled, or after removing visible material with soap and water, decontaminate hands with alcohol-based hand rub. Alternatively, hands may be washed with an antimicrobial soap and water.

Perform Hand Hygiene:
- Before having direct contact with patients
- After contact with blood, body fluids, or excretions, mucous membranes, non-intact skin, or wound dressings
- After contact with a patient's intact skin (e.g. when taking a pulse or blood pressure or lifting a patient)
- If hands will be moving from a contaminated body site to a clean body site during patient care
- After contact with inanimate objects (including medical equipment) in the immediate vicinity of the patient
- After removing gloves

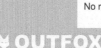

Patient Transport

Limit transport and movement of patients to medically-necessary purposes.

If transport or movement in any healthcare setting is necessary, instruct patient to wear a mask and follow Respiratory Hygiene/Cough Etiquette.

No mask is required for persons transporting patients on Droplet Precautions.

OUTFOX PREVENTION
www.OUTFOXprevention.com

OPDP1 ©2012 OUTFOX Prevention

Source: CDC/Centers for Disease Control and Prevention.

Figure B-5
Droplet precautions.

DROPLET PRECAUTIONS
From: 2007 Guideline for Isolation Precautions: Preventing Transmission of Infectious Agents in Healthcare Settings

V.C.   Droplet Precautions

V.C.1. Use Droplet Precautions as recommended in Appendix A for patients known or suspected to be infected with pathogens transmitted by respiratory droplets (i.e., large-particle droplets >5 in size) that are generated by a patient who is coughing, sneezing or talking.

V.C.2. Patient placement

V.C.2.a. In acute care hospitals, place patients who require Droplet Precautions in a single-patient room when available. When single-patient rooms are in short supply, apply the following principles for making decisions on patient placement:

-Prioritize patients who have excessive cough and sputum production for single-patient room placement

-Place together in the same room (cohort) patients who are infected the same pathogen and are suitable roommates.

-If it becomes necessary to place patients who require Droplet Precautions in a room with a patient who does not have the same infection:

-Avoid placing patients on Droplet Precautions in the same room with patients who have conditions that may increase the risk of adverse outcome from infection or that may facilitate transmission (e.g., those who are immunocompromised, have or have anticipated prolonged lengths of stay).

-Ensure that patients are physically separated (i.e., >3 feet apart) from each other. Draw the privacy curtain between beds to minimize opportunities for close contact.

-Change protective attire and perform hand hygiene between contact with patients in the same room, regardless of whether one patient or both patients are on Droplet Precautions.

V.C.2.b. In *long-term care and other residential settings*, make decisions regarding patient placement on a case-by-case basis after considering infection risks to other patients in the room and available alternatives.

V.C.2.c. In *ambulatory settings*, place patients who require Droplet Precautions in an examination room or cubicle as soon as possible. Instruct patients to follow recommendations for Respiratory Hygiene/Cough Etiquette.

V.C.3. Use of personal protective equipment

V.C.3.a. Don a mask upon entry into the patient room or cubicle.

V.C.3.b. No recommendation for routinely wearing eye protection (e.g., goggle or face shield), in addition to a mask, for close contact with patients who require Droplet Precautions. *Unresolved issue*

V.C.3.c. For patients with suspected or proven SARS, avian influenza or pandemic influenza, refer to the following websites for the most current recommendations (www.cdc.gov/ncidod/sars/ ; www.cdc.gov/flu/avian/ ; www.pandemicflu.gov/)

V.C.4. Patient transport

V.C.4.a. In *acute care hospitals and long-term care and other residential settings*, limit transport and movement of patients outside of the room to medically-necessary purposes.

V.C.4.b. If transport or movement in any healthcare setting is necessary, instruct patient to wear a mask and follow Respiratory Hygiene/Cough Etiquette www.cdc.gov/flu/professionals/infectioncontrol/resphygiene.htm).

V.C.4.c. No mask is required for persons transporting patients on Droplet Precautions.

V.C.4.d. Discontinue Droplet Precautions after signs and symptoms have resolved or according to pathogen-specific recommendations in Appendix A.

OPDP1 ©2012 OUTFOX Prevention

Figure B-5
(continued)

RESPIRATORY INFECTION ETIQUETTE

ATTENTION!

ATTENTION! **VISITORS,** please inform a staff member if you have signs or symptoms of any respiratory infection. In addition, please adhere to the following:

Cover:
-Use a tissue or the crook of the elbow during a cough or a sneeze.
-Despite covering during coughs and sneezes, sit at least 3 feet away from other people.
-Dispose of used tissues or wash unclean clothing as soon as possible.

Wash:
Wash all objects and clothing that could have been contaminated with the associated respiratory infection.
-Wash hands by performing effective hand hygiene:
        -Wash with warm water and soap
        -OR use an alcohol based hand sanitizer
        -OR use an antiseptic hand wash

Wear:
Wear a mask to minimize the distance that secretions may travel. Wear a mask as much as possible and not just during a cough or sneeze. Dispose of the mask after use.

Alert:
Alert a staff member if you have signs or symptoms of any respiratory infection. Suggest adhering to certain precautions from the Standard Precautions (i.e. Droplet Precautions, Contact Precautions, Airborne Precautions, etc.)

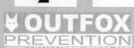

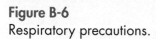

OUTFOX PREVENTION
www.OUTFOXprevention.com

OPRIE1 ©2010 OUTFOX Prevention

Figure B-6
Respiratory precautions.

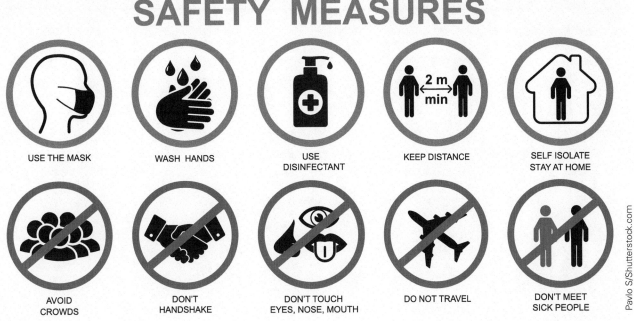

Figure B-7
COVID-19 safety measures.

Appendix C

Vital Signs

Table C-1
Body Temperature

	Oral	Axillary	Rectal
Average (normal temperature)	98.6°F (37°C)	97.6°F (36.5°C)	99.6°F (37.5°C)
Range	97.6–99.6°F (36.5–37.5°C)	96.6–98°F (36–37°C)	98.6–100.6°F (37–38.1°C)

Table C-2
Pulse Rate

Age	Pulse Rate in Beats per Minute
Less than 1 year	100–160
1–10 years	70–120
11–Adult years	60–100
Midlife adult	60–100
Older adult	60–80
Conditioned athlete	40–60

Table C-3
Blood Pressure

Blood Pressure Classification	Systolic Blood Pressure (mm Hg)	Diastolic Blood Pressure (mm Hg)
Normal	<120	and <80
Prehypertension	120–139	or 85–89
Stage 1 hypertension	140–159	or 90–99
Stage 2 hypertension	≥160	or ≥100

Table C-4
Respiration Rate

Age Category	Rate in Breaths per Minute
Newborn	30–60
Early childhood	20–40
Late childhood	16–26
Adults (16 years and older)	16–20

Appendix D

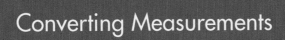

Converting Measurements

Length	Centimeters	inches	Feet
1 centimeter	1.000	0.394	0.0328
1 inch	2.54	1.000	0.0833
1 foot	30.48	12.000	1.000
1 yard	91.4	36.00	3.00
1 meter	100.00	39.40	3.28

Volumes	Cubic Centimeters	Fluid Drams	Fluid Ounces	Quarts	Liters
1 cubic centimeter	1.00	0.270	0.033	0.0010	0.0010
1 fluid dram	3.70	1.00	0.125	0.0039	0.0037
1 cubic inch	16.39	4.43	0.554	0.0173	0.0163
1 fluid ounce	29.6	8.00	1.000	0.0312	0.0296
1 quart	946.0	255.0	32.00	1.000	0.946
1 liter	1,000.0	270.0	33.80	1.056	1.000

Weights	Grains	Grams	Apothecary Ounces	Pounds
1 grain (gr)	1.000	0.064	0.002	0.0001
1 gram (g)	15.43	1.000	0.032	0.0022
1 apothecary ounce	480.00	31.1	1.000	0.0685
1 pound	7,000.00	454.0	14.58	1.000
1 kilogram	15,432.0	1,000.00	32.15	2.205

Rules for Converting One System to Another

Volumes

Grains to grams—divide by 15
Drams to cubic centimeters—multiply by 4
Ounces to cubic centimeters—multiply by 30
Minims to cubic millimeters—multiply by 63
Minims to cubic centimeters—multiply by 0.06
Cubic millimeters to minims—divide by 63
Cubic centimeters to minims—multiply by 16
Cubic centimeters to fluid ounces—divide by 30
Liters to pints—divide by 2.1

Weights

Pounds to kilograms—divide by 2.2
Kilograms to pounds—multiply by 2.2
Milligrams to grains—multiply by 0.0154
Grams to grains—multiply by 15
Grams to drams—multiply by 0.257
Grams to ounces—multiply by 0.0311

Temperature

Multiply centigrade (Celsius) degrees by $\frac{9}{5}$ and add 32 to convert Fahrenheit to Celsius.
Subtract 32 from the Fahrenheit degrees and multiply by $\frac{5}{9}$ to convert Celsius to Fahrenheit.

Common Household Measures

1 teaspoon = 4–5 mL or 1 dram
3 teaspoons = 1 tablespoon
1 dessert spoon = 8 mL or 2 drams
1 tablespoon = 15 mL or 3 drams
4 tablespoons = 1 wine glass or ½ gill
16 tablespoons (liq) = 1 cup
12 tablespoons (dry) = 1 cup
1 cup = 8 fluid ounces or ½ pint
1 tumbler or glass = 8 fluid ounces or 240 mL
1 wine glass = 2 fluid ounces, 60 mL
16 fluid ounces = 1 pound
4 gills = 1 pound
1 pint = 1 pound

Appendix E

Medical Terminology

Table E–1
Common Combining Forms That Refer to Body Parts

Combining Form	Meaning	Combining Form	Meaning
adip/o; lip/o; steat/o	fat	lapar/o	abdominal wall
arteri/o	artery	laryng/o	voice box, larynx
arthr/o	joint	myel/o	spinal cord
axill/o	armpit	my/o; muscul/o	muscle
blephar/o	eyelid	nas/o; rhin/o	nose
cardi/o	heart	neur/o	nerve
cephal/o	head	ophthalm/o; ocul/o	eye
cerebr/o; encephal/o	cerebrum, brain	or/o; stomat/o	mouth
cervic/o	neck	oste/o	bone
cholecyst/o	gallbladder	ot/o	ear
col/o	large intestine	pancreat/o	pancreas
cost/o	rib	pharyng/o	throat
crani/o	skull	pneum/o; pneumon/o	lung
cyst/o	urinary bladder	ren/o; nephr/o	kidneys
cyt/o	cell	splen/o	spleen
derm/o; dermat/o	skin	thorac/o	chest
enter/o	small intestine	thyroid/o	thyroid gland
esophag/o	esophagus	trache/o	windpipe, trachea
gastr/o	stomach	ven/o; phleb/o	vein
hem/o; hemat/o	blood	vertebr/o	vertebra
hepat/o	liver		

Table E–2
Color Word Roots

Word Root	Meaning	Example
cyan/o	blue	cyanosis (sigh ah NOH sis) blueish discoloration of the skin
erythr/o	red	erythrocyte (eh RITH roh sight) red blood cell
leuk/o	white	leukocyte (LOO koh sight)
melan/o	black	melanoma (mel uh NO muh) tumor of melanin-forming cells (melanin is a dark brown or black pigment)
poli/o	gray	poliomyelitis (poh lee oh my eh LIE tis) infection of the gray nerve tissue of the spinal cord

Table E–3
Common Suffixes

Suffix	Meaning	Term	Meaning
-ac, -al, -ar, -ary, -eal, -ia, -iac, -ic, -ical, -ose, -ous, -tic	All of these mean "pertaining to"	cardi**ac** cellul**ar** psycho**tic**	pertaining to the heart pertaining to the cell pertaining to psychosis
-algia	pain, painful condition	neur**algia** (new RAL jee ah)	pain along a nerve
-centesis	surgical puncture to remove fluid	amnio**centesis** (am nee oh sin TEE sis)	insertion of needle to withdraw sample of amniotic fluid
-cide	to kill, destroy	germi**cide** (JER mih side)	chemical substance that kills germs
-cyte	cell	leuko**cyte** (LOO koh cite)	white blood cell
-ectomy	surgical removal of	gastr**ectomy** (gas TREK toh me)	removal of part or all of the stomach
-emia	blood; blood condition	bacter**emia** (back ter EE mee ah)	bacteria in the blood
-gram	record	electrocardio**gram** (ee lek troh KAR dee oh gram)	record of the electrical activity of the heart
-graph	an instrument used to record	electrocardio**graph** (ee lek troh KAR dee ah graf)	instrument that records electrical variations in cardiac muscle activity
-graphy	process of recording	electrocardio**graphy** (ee lek troh kar dee AH graf ee)	the making and study of electrocardiograms
-ia	condition, especially an abnormal state	tachycard**ia** (tak ee KAR dee ah)	condition of abnormal rapid heart rate
-ion	condition	hypertens**ion** (high per TEN shun)	high blood pressure

(continues)

Table E–3 (continued)

Suffix	Meaning	Term	Meaning
-ism	condition	hypothyroid**ism** (high poh THIGH roid izm)	condition created by less than normal levels of thyroid hormones
-itis	inflammation of	card**itis** (kar DYE tis)	inflammation of the heart
-lithiasis	presence of or formation of stones	chole**lithiasis** (koh lee lih THIGH ah sis)	presence of stones in the gallbladder
-logy	study of	cardio**logy** (kar dee OL oh jee)	study of the heart
-megaly	enlargement	hepato**megaly** (hep ah toh MEG ah lee)	enlargement of the liver
-oid	resembling	rheumat**oid** (ROO mah toyd)	resembling rheumatism
-oma	tumor	my**oma** (my OH mah)	tumor containing muscle tissue
-osis	abnormal condition or disease	nephr**osis** (nef ROH sis)	kidney disease
-otomy	surgical incision	trache**otomy** (tray kee OT oh mee)	incision into trachea
-pathy	disease	encephalo**pathy** (en sef ah LOP ah thee)	disease of the brain
-plasty	surgical or plastic repair	rhino**plasty** (RYE no plas tee)	plastic surgery of the nose
-plegia	paralysis	hemi**plegia** (hem ee PLEE jee ah)	paralysis of one side (half) of the body
-pnea	breathing, respiration	a**pnea** (ap NEE ah)	temporary cessation of breathing
-rrhaphy	surgical suturing	gastro**rrhaphy** (gas TROR uh fee)	suturing a perforation of the stomach
-rrhea	drainage, flow, discharge	rhino**rrhea** (rye no REE ah)	drainage from the nose
-rrhexis	rupture	cardio**rrhexis** (car dee oh REX is)	rupture of the heart wall
-scope	instrument used to view	oto**scope** (OH toh skope)	instrument used to examine the ear
-scopy	examination using a scope	sigmoido**scopy** (sig moy DOS koh pee)	examination of the sigmoid colon using a scope
-sis	action, process, state, condition	myco**sis** (my COH sis)	disease caused by a fungus
-stasis	stoppage, controlling, standing	veno**stasis** (vee no STAY sis)	stoppage of blood in a vein
-stomy	surgically create an artificial mouth or stoma (opening)	colo**stomy** (koh LOSS toh me)	surgical opening into the colon to create a stoma

Table E–4
Common Prefixes

Prefix	Meaning	Term	Meaning
a-/an-	without, not, absence of	**an**uria (an YOU ree ah)	absence of urine formation
anti-	against	**an**tibiotic (an tie buy AHT ick)	substance that inhibits growth of or destroys microorganisms
auto-	self	**auto**immune (aw toh ih MYOON)	disease that results in immune response to one's own body
bi-	two, double	**bi**furcate (BUY fur kate)	having two branches or divisions
brady-	slow	**brady**cardia (brad ee KAR dee ah)	slow heart rate
dys-	bad, difficult, painful, abnormal	**dys**pnea (disp NEE ah)	difficulty breathing
epi-	over, above, upon	**epi**gastric (ep ih GAS trik)	over the stomach
eu-	good, normal	**eu**pnea (yoop NEE ah)	normal breathing
hemi-	half	**hemi**plegia (hem ee PLEE jee ah)	paralysis of one side or half of the body
hyper-	above, excessive	**hyper**tension (high per TEN shun)	high blood pressure
hypo-	less than, under	**hypo**tension (high poh TEN shun)	low blood pressure
inter-	between	**inter**costal (in ter COS tahl)	between the ribs
intra-	within	**intra**venous (in trah VEE nus)	within a vein
multi-	many	**multi**nodal (mul tee NO dahl)	having many nodes or knots
non-	not	**non**toxic (non TOK sik)	not poisonous
peri-	around, surrounding	**peri**anal (per ee A nal)	around the anus
poly-	many, much	**poly**uria (pol ee YOU ree ah)	excretion of large amounts of urine
post-	after, behind	**post**operative (post OP er ah tiv)	following a surgical procedure
pre-	before, in front	**pre**operative (pree OP er ah tiv)	before a surgical procedure
pseudo-	false	**pseudo**hematuria (sue doh hee mah TOO ree ah)	red pigment in the urine that makes the urine "falsely" appear to have blood in it
quadri-	four	**quadri**plegia (kwad rih PLEE jee ah)	paralysis of all four extremities
semi-	half	**semi**permeable (sem ee PER mee ah bull)	half permeable—a membrane that allows fluids but not the dissolved substance to pass through
sub-	under, below	**sub**sternal (sub STIR nuhl)	below the sternum
supra-	above, over	**supra**pubic (sue prah PEW bik)	above the pubic area
tachy-	fast, rapid	**tachy**cardia (tak ee KAR dee ah)	rapid heart rate
tri-	three	**tri**chotomy (try COT oh me)	division into three parts

Table E–5
Medical Terminology and Abbreviations

Abbreviation	Meaning	Abbreviation	Meaning
a	before	mEq	milliequivalent
ac	before meals	mg	milligram
AD	right ear	ml, mL	milliliter (equivalent to cc)
AM, am	morning	mm	millimeter
AS	left ear	NEB	nebulizer
AU	both ears	NG	nasogastric
bid	twice a day	NPO, npo	nothing by mouth
cap	capsule	NS, N/S, NSS	normal saline (sodium chloride, 0.9%)
cm	centimeter	OD	right eye
c̄	with	ODT	orally disintegrating tablet
D/C, dc	discontinue	OS	left eye
D5W	dextrose 5% in water	OU	both eyes
DS	double strength	oz	ounce
EC	enteric coated	p	after
ER	extended release	pc	after meals
g, gm	gram	PM, pm	afternoon
gr	grains	po, PO	by mouth, orally
gtt	drop	PRN, prn	whenever necessary or as needed
h, hr	hour	q2h	every 2 hours
Hs	bedtime	qh	every hour
IM	intramuscular	qid	four times a day
IV	intravenous	qs	quantity sufficient
IVPB	intravenous piggyback	R, pr	rectal, per rectum
kg, Kilo	kilogram	RL, R/L	Ringer's lactate
KVO	keep vein open	s̄	without
LA	long acting	sc/subcuᵃ	subcutaneous
L	liter	SL	sublingual
LR	lactated Ringer's	SR	sustained release
mcg	microgram	stat	immediately and once only
supp	suppository	TO	telephone order
tab	tablet	tsp, t	teaspoon
tbsp, T, tbs	tablespoon	Vag/PV	vaginal
tid	three times daily	VO	verbal order

Note: Abbreviations should be written without periods. Also some abbreviations in this table are on the ISMP's List of Error-Prone Abbreviations, Symbols, and Dose Designations, but it is still important to know them.

ᵃ Although subcutaneous can also have the abbreviations of SC, SQ, or subq, these abbreviations are noted on the ISMP's List of Error-Prone Abbreviations, Symbols, and Dose Designations. When handwritten, they can be confused for other terms. Therefore, we will be using "subcu" throughout the chapters. With the expected near-future universal implementation of electronic records and electronic charting, handwritten look-alike errors will hopefully become a thing of the past.

ISMP's List of *Error-Prone Abbreviations, Symbols,* and *Dose Designations*

The abbreviations, symbols, and dose designations found in this table have been reported to ISMP through the ISMP National Medication Errors Reporting Program (ISMP MERP) as being frequently misinterpreted and involved in harmful medication errors. They should **NEVER** be used when communicating medical information. This includes internal communications, telephone/verbal prescriptions, computer-generated labels, labels for drug storage bins, medication administration records, as well as pharmacy and prescriber computer order entry screens.

Abbreviations	Intended Meaning	Misinterpretation	Correction
μg	Microgram	Mistaken as "mg"	Use "mcg"
AD, AS, AU	Right ear, left ear, each ear	Mistaken as OD, OS, OU (right eye, left eye, each eye)	Use "right ear," "left ear," or "each ear"
OD, OS, OU	Right eye, left eye, each eye	Mistaken as AD, AS, AU (right ear, left ear, each ear)	Use "right eye," "left eye," or "each eye"
BT	Bedtime	Mistaken as "BID" (twice daily)	Use "bedtime"
cc	Cubic centimeters	Mistaken as "u" (units)	Use "mL"
D/C	Discharge or discontinue	Premature discontinuation of medications if D/C (intended to mean "discharge") has been misinterpreted as "discontinued" when followed by a list of discharge medications	Use "discharge" and "discontinue"
IJ	Injection	Mistaken as "IV" or "intrajugular"	Use "injection"
IN	Intranasal	Mistaken as "IM" or "IV"	Use "intranasal" or "NAS"
HS	Half-strength	Mistaken as bedtime	Use "half-strength" or "bedtime"
hs	At bedtime, hours of sleep	Mistaken as half-strength	
IU**	International unit	Mistaken as IV (intravenous) or 10 (ten)	Use "units"
o.d. or OD	Once daily	Mistaken as "right eye" (OD-oculus dexter), leading to oral liquid medications administered in the eye	Use "daily"
OJ	Orange juice	Mistaken as OD or OS (right or left eye); drugs meant to be diluted in orange juice may be given in the eye	Use "orange juice"
Per os	By mouth, orally	The "os" can be mistaken as "left eye" (OS-oculus sinister)	Use "PO," "by mouth," or "orally"
q.d. or QD**	Every day	Mistaken as q.i.d., especially if the period after the "q" or the tail of the "q" is misunderstood as an "i"	Use "daily"
qhs	Nightly at bedtime	Mistaken as "qhr" or every hour	Use "nightly"
qn	Nightly or at bedtime	Mistaken as "qh" (every hour)	Use "nightly" or "at bedtime"
q.o.d. or QOD**	Every other day	Mistaken as "q.d." (daily) or "q.i.d. (four times daily) if the "o" is poorly written	Use "every other day"
q1d	Daily	Mistaken as q.i.d. (four times daily)	Use "daily"
q6PM, etc.	Every evening at 6 PM	Mistaken as every 6 hours	Use "daily at 6 PM" or "6 PM daily"
SC, SQ, sub q	Subcutaneous	SC mistaken as SL (sublingual); SQ mistaken as "5 every;" the "q" in "sub q" has been mistaken as "every" (e.g., a heparin dose ordered "sub q 2 hours before surgery" misunderstood as every 2 hours before surgery)	Use "subcut" or "subcutaneously"
ss	Sliding scale (insulin) or ½ (apothecary)	Mistaken as "55"	Spell out "sliding scale;" use "one-half" or "½"
SSRI	Sliding scale regular insulin	Mistaken as selective-serotonin reuptake inhibitor	Spell out "sliding scale (insulin)"
SSI	Sliding scale insulin	Mistaken as Strong Solution of Iodine (Lugol's)	
i/d	One daily	Mistaken as "tid"	Use "1 daily"
TIW or tiw	3 times a week	Mistaken as "3 times a day" or "twice in a week"	Use "3 times weekly"
U or u**	Unit	Mistaken as the number 0 or 4, causing a 10-fold overdose or greater (e.g., 4U seen as "40" or 4u seen as "44"); mistaken as "cc" so dose given in volume instead of units (e.g., 4u seen as 4cc)	Use "unit"
UD	As directed ("ut dictum")	Mistaken as unit dose (e.g., diltiazem 125 mg IV infusion "UD" misinterpreted as meaning to give the entire infusion as a unit [bolus] dose)	Use "as directed"

ISMP's List of *Error-Prone Abbreviations, Symbols,* and *Dose Designations* (continued)

Dose Designations and Other Information	Intended Meaning	Misinterpretation	Correction
Trailing zero after decimal point (e.g., 1.0 mg)**	1 mg	Mistaken as 10 mg if the decimal point is not seen	Do not use trailing zeros for doses expressed in whole numbers
"Naked" decimal point (e.g., .5 mg)**	0.5 mg	Mistaken as 5 mg if the decimal point is not seen	Use zero before a decimal point when the dose is less than a whole unit
Abbreviations such as mg. or mL. with a period following the abbreviation	mg mL	The period is unnecessary and could be mistaken as the number 1 if written poorly	Use mg, mL, etc. without a terminal period

Dose Designations and Other Information	Intended Meaning	Misinterpretation	Correction
Drug name and dose run together (especially problematic for drug names that end in "l" such as Inderal40 mg; Tegretol300 mg)	Inderal 40 mg Tegretol 300 mg	Mistaken as Inderal 140 mg Mistaken as Tegretol 1300 mg	Place adequate space between the drug name, dose, and unit of measure
Numerical dose and unit of measure run together (e.g., 10mg, 100mL)	10 mg 100 mL	The "m" is sometimes mistaken as a zero or two zeros, risking a 10- to 100-fold overdose	Place adequate space between the dose and unit of measure
Large doses without properly placed commas (e.g., 100000 units; 1000000 units)	100,000 units 1,000,000 units	100000 has been mistaken as 10,000 or 1,000,000; 1000000 has been mistaken as 100,000	Use commas for dosing units at or above 1,000, or use words such as 100 "thousand" or 1 "million" to improve readability

Drug Name Abbreviations	Intended Meaning	Misinterpretation	Correction
To avoid confusion, do not abbreviate drug names when communicating medical information. Examples of drug name abbreviations involved in medication errors include:			
APAP	acetaminophen	Not recognized as acetaminophen	Use complete drug name
ARA A	vidarabine	Mistaken as cytarabine (ARA C)	Use complete drug name
AZT	zidovudine (Retrovir)	Mistaken as azathioprine or aztreonam	Use complete drug name
CPZ	Compazine (prochlorperazine)	Mistaken as chlorpromazine	Use complete drug name
DPT	Demerol-Phenergan-Thorazine	Mistaken as diphtheria-pertussis-tetanus (vaccine)	Use complete drug name
DTO	Diluted tincture of opium, or deodorized tincture of opium (Paregoric)	Mistaken as tincture of opium	Use complete drug name
HCl	hydrochloric acid or hydrochloride	Mistaken as potassium chloride (The "H" is misinterpreted as "K")	Use complete drug name unless expressed as a salt of a drug
HCT	hydrocortisone	Mistaken as hydrochlorothiazide	Use complete drug name
HCTZ	hydrochlorothiazide	Mistaken as hydrocortisone (seen as HCT250 mg)	Use complete drug name
MgSO4**	magnesium sulfate	Mistaken as morphine sulfate	Use complete drug name
MS, MSO4**	morphine sulfate	Mistaken as magnesium sulfate	Use complete drug name
MTX	methotrexate	Mistaken as mitoxantrone	Use complete drug name
PCA	procainamide	Mistaken as patient controlled analgesia	Use complete drug name
PTU	propylthiouracil	Mistaken as mercaptopurine	Use complete drug name
T3	Tylenol with codeine No. 3	Mistaken as liothyronine	Use complete drug name
TAC	triamcinolone	Mistaken as tetracaine, Adrenalin, cocaine	Use complete drug name
TNK	TNKase	Mistaken as "TPA"	Use complete drug name
ZnSO4	zinc sulfate	Mistaken as morphine sulfate	Use complete drug name

ISMP's List of *Error-Prone Abbreviations, Symbols,* and *Dose Designations* (continued)

Stemmed Drug Names	Intended Meaning	Misinterpretation	Correction
"Nitro" drip	nitroglycerin infusion	Mistaken as sodium nitroprusside infusion	Use complete drug name
"Norflox"	norfloxacin	Mistaken as Norflex	Use complete drug name
"IV Vanc"	intravenous vancomycin	Mistaken as Invanz	Use complete drug name

Symbols	Intended Meaning	Misinterpretation	Correction
ʒ	Dram	Symbol for dram mistaken as "3"	Use the metric system
♏	Minim	Symbol for minim mistaken as "mL"	
x3d	For three days	Mistaken as "3 doses"	Use "for three days"
> and <	Greater than and less than	Mistaken as opposite of intended; mistakenly use incorrect symbol; "< 10" mistaken as "40"	Use "greater than" or "less than"
/ (slash mark)	Separates two doses or indicates "per"	Mistaken as the number 1 (e.g., "25 units/10 units" misread as "25 units and 110" units)	Use "per" rather than a slash mark to separate doses
@	At	Mistaken as "2"	Use "at"
&	And	Mistaken as "2"	Use "and"
+	Plus or and	Mistaken as "4"	Use "and"
°	Hour	Mistaken as a zero (e.g., q2° seen as q 20)	Use "hr," "h," or "hour"
Φ or ⊘	zero, null sign	Mistaken as numerals 4, 6, 8, and 9	Use 0 or zero, or describe intent using whole words

**These abbreviations are included on The Joint Commission's "minimum list" of dangerous abbreviations, acronyms, and symbols that must be included on an organization's "Do Not Use" list, effective January 1, 2004. Visit www.jointcommission.org for more information about this Joint Commission requirement.

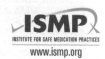

ISMP
INSTITUTE FOR SAFE MEDICATION PRACTICES
www.ismp.org

Appendix F

Answers to Select Feature Boxes

Only feature boxes which have distinct, specific answers are included in this appendix. Other feature boxes are designed for self-reflection and in-class discussion.

Chapter 1

Skill Application 1-4: Helping Memory Skills

1. PAIL
2. SOAP
3. SOAPIE

Just for Fun 1-1: Acronyms and Mnemonics

Answers: (these are just suggestions; you can come up with your own as well)

1. Every Good Boy Does Fine
2. Richard Of York Got Buggered In Venice or ROY G. BIV
3. To Pass Right Behind

Chapter 2

Just for Fun 2-1: A Look at Idioms

Answers:

1. c
2. f
3. j
4. b
5. h
6. g
7. a
8. e
9. d
10. i

Chapter 3

Test Yourself 3-1: Which Is a Better Goal?

Answers:

1. B
2. A
3. A
4. A
5. A

Just for Fun 3-1: Prioritizing Tasks

Answers: (there are other possible orderings as long as no time conflicts occur)

7   Do afternoon treatment rounds (1300 to 1430).

10   Research at the library for a report to your medical director due in 2 weeks.

4   Reserve a conference room for an in-service for your department. This must be done by 1100.

1   Do morning treatment rounds (0715 to 0915).

2   Call two home care patients to reschedule appointments for tomorrow.

5   Fix and calibrate equipment in the utility room. This will take about 1 hour.

9   Complete billing charges for yesterday—must be done by end of shift and will take about 30 minutes.

6   Eat lunch with medical equipment salesperson.

8   Give end-of-shift report to oncoming 1500 to 2300 shift (about 30 minutes).

3   Scheduled meeting from 0930 to 1000 with department director concerning my upcoming promotion and raise for doing such a professional job.

Chapter 4

Just for Fun 4-1: Mental Gymnastics

Answers:

King is smaller than both the dog and Rover. Therefore, King is the cat because that is the only animal smaller than the dog, assuming that a goat and a horse would be bigger than even a big cat.

The horse is younger than Angel or Beauty. Therefore, the horse is Rover because it cannot be Angel, Beauty, or King.

Beauty is the oldest and a good friend of the dog. Therefore, Beauty is not the dog and must then be the goat. This leaves the dog being Angel.

Test Yourself 4-1: Facts Concerning Creativity

Answers:

1. False

Highly intelligent people may have a tendency to not think up new ideas; however, they may be very analytical in dealing with established concepts. In essence, they may think they know *all* the answers and not be open to new ones. Many creative individuals throughout history had IQ scores in the normal range.

2. False

Although the computer will help us process information faster, as of yet, it will not think for us or generate a totally independent idea outside of the programming we humans put in.

3. True

Fear of failure prevents you from taking mental risks and thinking outside the box. Fear of failure also impacts our self-esteem or our confidence in our ability to be creative.

Just for Fun 4-2: Brain Teasers

1. An electric train does not blow smoke.
2. A nickel and fifty-cent piece. We said one is not a nickel; the other one can be.
3. We have numbered the squares to give you the 30 combinations. Answer: First, there are the obvious 16 single squares; next is the one big square made from all the little squares combined. This brings us to 17 squares. The remaining combinations are as follows: There are 9 four-square combinations, bringing the total to 26.

1	2	3	4
5	6	7	8
9	10	11	12
13	14	15	16

1-2-5-6, 2-3-6-7, 3-4-7-8, 5-6-9-10, 6-7-10-11, 7-8-11-12, 9-10-13-14, 10-11-14-15, 11-12-15-16.

There are 4 nine-square combinations, bringing the total to 30.

1-2-3-5-6-7-9-10-11, 2-3-4-6-7-8-10-11-12, 5-6-7-9-10-11-13-14-15, 6-7-8-10-11-12-14-15-16.

Just for Fun 4-3: Mental Flexibility

Answers:

26 Letters of the Alphabet

12 Signs of the Zodiac

52 Cards in a Deck without Jokers

8 Planets in the Solar System (there is still controversy about Pluto being a planet so this one might stir debate)

88 Piano Keys

18 Holes on a Golf Course

29 Days in February in a Leap Year

206 Bones in the Body

4 Quarts in a Gallon

2 Pints in a Quart

8 Sides on a Stop Sign

Just for Fun 4-4: Do Not Be Afraid to Color Outside the Lines

Answers:

Solution to connect all the nine dots with four straight lines without lifting the pencil from the paper.

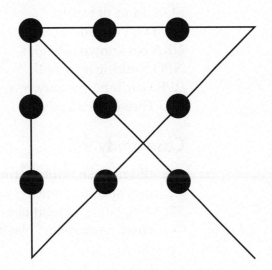

Chapter 7

Just for Fun 7-1: Many Meanings
Answers:

1. E
2. B
3. G
4. D
5. A
6. F
7. C

Chapter 9

Test Yourself 9-1: Medical Lingo
Answers:

STAT Immediately
MOM Milk of Magnesia
BID Twice daily
PRN As needed
SOB Short of breath
OOB Out of bed
NKA No known allergies
NPO Nothing by mouth
CPR Cardiopulmonary resuscitation
TID Three times daily

Case Study 9-1

1. did not use military time
2. non-specific time
3. derogatory patient comment
4. charting someone else's work

Chapter 11

Test Yourself 11-1: Negligence or Malpractice

1. negligence
2. malpractice
3. negligence
4. malpractice

Glossary

abandonment leaving a patient who needs additional care

acronym a word made from the first letter of other words

active listening when the mind is focusing on both the message and the speaker during the communication process

active reader One who reads with determination to understand and critically think about what they are reading

advance directive document stating the patient's wishes concerning the handling of their body while the person is still living

advocating speaking or acting on behalf of a patient who may not be able to or know how to do so for themselves

affective domain one area of learning identified in Bloom's taxonomy concerning behavioral learning. This domain deals with attitudes, motivation, willingness to learn and participate, and professionalism.

against medical advice (AMA) when a patient insists on leaving the health care institution and has been advised against leaving and told of the dangers of disrupting treatment

airborne precautions set of precautions for airborne spread infection

analogy forces cross-connections between two unlike things

assertive a confident personality that uses "I" messages and demands to be heard without using anger or blaming

asynchronous distance education a type of distance education in which the teacher and student interact from different places and times

bad stress when anxiety reaches a level that interferes with performance or stops performance entirely

battery the use of touch or force without the patient's consent

behavioral interview a type of job interview in which the applicant is asked to describe behaviors or situations. The interviewer is looking for a "fit" with the hiring institution. For example, "Tell me about a time when you faced a difficult patient and how you handled it."

brain death irreversible cessation of all functions of the brain

brainstorming when a group of people get together and come up with ideas concerning an opportunity or issue

brand Features, characteristics, and/or traits that define you and your unique story

caring attitude sincerity, empathy, respect, and consideration toward others

certification the result of a formal process of identifying and acknowledging individuals who have successfully completed or attained some level of excellence, often the result of passing a standardized examination

chain of infection a term that defines the source of infection, continues with the transportation of the infection, and ends with the entry into the body. Breaking any of the links of the chain can interrupt the infectious process.

charting the process of recording information on a patient's chart; the chart is a legal document that includes confidential material on patient history, current medical status, and recovery process.

chief complaint/chief concern (CC) the patient's main reason for seeking medical help

classical conditioning repeated actions that lead to a desired behavior

classroom etiquette behaviors and actions that are appropriate, acceptable, and desired in the classroom setting

clear message a message that delivers the intended meaning

close-ended questions questions that can be answered with a simple yes or no response

cognitive domain one area of learning identified in Bloom's taxonomy. This domain focuses on intellectual skills.

cognitive processes the complex mental activities that constitute thinking

cohesiveness the degree to which members work together

colloquial language informal words and phrases such as "sleep tight" or "don't cause a ruckus." Informal language should not be used when communicating with patients.

communication the exchange of messages, information, thoughts, ideas, and feelings

communication process the process of communicating, which includes a sender presenting a clear message to a receiver who relays feedback

competency being capable of doing something well

complacency an interference during the communication process that results in the message getting through but is being acted on only half-heartedly or not at all

confidentiality keeping personal information such as health information private

conformity changing one's opinion or behavior in response to pressure from a group

constructive concern converting useless worries into positive improvements

contact precautions set of precautions for infections spread by contact

continuing education instructional programs taken to keep participants up-to-date and current in a particular area of knowledge

continuing education credits credits earned after successful participation in continuing education activities such as attending a conference or webinar

cover letter accompanies a résumé and helps demonstrate interest in the job that is being sought by getting the attention of the employer

creative thinking the generation of ideas that results in the improvement of the efficiency or the effectiveness of the system

critical thinking the ability to gather and analyze information to solve problems or create new opportunities

cultural competence the combination of knowledge, belief, and behavior that has a positive effect on patient care by allowing providers to deliver care that is respectful to the beliefs and practices of all patients regardless of culture

customer relations refers to the way clients (patients and visitors) are treated by the employees of a business

decision making the act of making an informed choice between a number of alternatives in order to solve a problem and/or maximize an opportunity

decodes the receiver interprets the message

deductive reasoning a form of logical thinking in which a true conclusion is based on true facts called premises

dependability the characteristics of being trustworthy and reliable; doing what you say you will do when you say you will do it

depression remaining sad for prolonged periods, which interferes with the ability to perform daily activities

diagonal communication the flow of communication between departments or people that are on different lateral planes of the organizational chart

dialysis medical treatment to assist your body in removal of extra fluid and waste products when the kidneys are not able to perform this function

directed thinking a conscious effort made to solve a specific problem or situation through learning, reasoning, and decision making

distance learning/education any learning that occurs through the Internet

distress anxiety

documentation the process of recording patient information, therapies, and responses

downward communication formal flow of communication from people with formal power to staff employees

droplet precautions set of precautions for infections spread by droplets, such as in a sneeze

durable medical equipment (DME) are supplies ordered by a health provider for extended and everyday use to improve the quality of life.

durable power of attorney a legal document that identifies another individual to make decisions for the patient if the patient is unable to

e-learning electronic learning as in online courses or webinars

elder abuse any knowing, intentional, or negligent act by a caregiver toward a vulnerable older adult

electronic communication communication via any electronic device (i.e., e-mail, text messaging, and FAX)

electronic health record (EHR) a digital version of a patient's paper health record. They are real-time, patient-centered, and shared among health care providers.

emotional intelligence (EI) being aware of, in control of, and able to monitor one's emotions

empathy the ability to feel and understand what others are going through

encoding the process of converting ideas or messages into words, diagrams, graphs, or reports

endorphins the body's natural painkillers

enunciation the clarity with which words are pronounced

environmental communication barriers when the environment interferes with the communication process

essay examination an exam that requires a narrative to answer the question

ethics conforming to accepted and professional standards of conduct

eustress normal stress that is interpreted as helpful

euthanasia medically assisting another to die

evidence-based practice applying the best available evidence, while taking patient preferences and clinical expertise into consideration, when making decisions in health care

false imprisonment restraining a person against their will

feedback information regarding a person's performance or ability

financial exploitation misusing the money or assets of another person in your care. A type of elder abuse.

formal communication channels communication flow that can be seen by viewing an organizational chart or flowchart that is established by the way the organization is put together

formal group a collection of people who share clear goals and expectations along with established rules of conduct

fraud consists of the intentional withholding or modification of information

functional résumé a list of one's experiences in terms of skills previously used on jobs or throughout one's educational career

goals specific accomplishments which one aims to achieve

good stress helps motivate a person to be up for a task

gossip mostly based on rumors and becomes more personal in nature; is usually directed at an individual or group of individuals

group dynamics the study of how people interact in groups

groupthink the unquestioning acceptance of the group's beliefs and behaviors

hand hygiene the appropriate use of hand-washing techniques

hand washing the most important step in preventing the spread of infection

health care proxy a legal document in which a person (patient) names another person to make health care decisions on their behalf if they are incapable of making health care decisions

Health Insurance Portability and Accountability Act (HIPAA) Federal legislation enacted in 1996 that established a well-defined set of regulations concerning protection of patient privacy

hearing the process, function, or power of perceiving sound; requires concentration while blocking out external and internal distractions

honesty telling the truth

horizontal communication when departments or groups of people on the same level of the organizational chart communicate with each other

hospice care a special part of the health care system that helps patients and their families throughout the grieving process and allows the patient to die with dignity, usually at home, where the patient feels most comfortable

immunologic pertaining to the immune system, which fights infections

inductive reasoning making the best guess based on premises or facts

infection control preventing health care associated infection

informal communication channels communication that is established through the "grapevine"

informal groups a loose association of people without stated rules or goals

informed consent any type of procedure requires that a patient sign a consent form stating that they have been instructed about what the procedure entails

inpatient a patient getting care while staying in the hospital

interview an evaluation of a potential employee's job skills, knowledge, character, and oral communication skills

intimate space the distance of 0 to 18 inches away from a patient

introductory stage the beginning of an interaction or relationship; with patients the introductory stage should take place within the social space of 4 to 12 feet

invasion of privacy any public discussion of private information concerning your patient

jargon words or expressions used by health care providers that are not understood by the general public

lateral communication communication at the same level of the organizational chart

lateral thinking a creative type of thinking that generates new ideas by connecting previously unrelated concepts

lay language words or terms understood by the general public

leadership a set of behaviors, attitudes, and values that enables the leader to motivate and direct others to act

license an official document that certifies your ability to practice your profession

licensure having a license to practice in the health care environment

lifelong learner a person who pursues education throughout their entire life in different times, places, and venues

line of authority the chain of command, usually found on an organizational chart that outlines the flow of communication for decision making

listening paying attention and focusing on the sounds that are heard

living will a written legal document that includes statements regarding health care wishes if you are no longer able to express yourself

logical thinking the ability to reason both deductively and inductively in a given situation

long-range goals goals to be accomplished within the next few years

malpractice any professional misconduct or lack of competency that results in injury to the patient

meditation focusing your attention while at the same time clearing your mind of thought

medium-range goals goals to be accomplished within the next six months to one year

mnemonics words, rhymes, or formulas that aid your memory

multicompetencies being competent in more than one area

multiskilling one person with multiple skills

negative attitude maintaining a pessimistic outlook during situations

negative pressure room a specialized room to prevent the spread of infections by venting the air to the outside

negligence the failure to give reasonable care; can be intentional or unintentional

nonrapid eye movement (NREM) sleep stages 1–3, characterized by decreased metabolic activity

nonverbal communication the use of behavior, such as facial expressions, gestures, body language, and touch to communicate

norms rules within particular groups that people in particular roles are expected to adhere to

objective the end task that is to be accomplished

objective examination an exam that has items such as multiple choice and true and false that require one answer

open-ended questions questions that require an explanation as a response

oral communication a form of verbal communication in which words are exchanged either face-to-face or through another means, such as a telephone

organizational chart a chart that shows the flow of communication, the relationships of various departments, and the lines of authority within an organization

outpatient receiving medical treatment without being admitted to the hospital overnight

palliative care a type of care provided during life-threatening illness that allows for advocacy, treatment of pain, and coordination of care

passive reader one who reads words without critically thinking

persistent vegetative state a patient who is completely unresponsive and being kept alive by medical intervention, irreversible

personal communication barriers when a problem exists within an individual or the person with whom the communication is taking place that interferes with the communication process

personal communication barriers personal characteristics that prevent effective communication, for example, certain attitudes, prejudices, or emotions that can interfere with the intended communication

personal protective equipment (PPE) specialized equipment to help stop the spread of infection, for example gloves, gowns, and masks

personal space the distance of approximately 18 inches to 4 feet away from a patient

physical abuse results from actual contact, usually resulting in a visible injury

plateau period period when little or no progress is made toward desired goals

positive attitude maintaining an optimistic outlook during situations

proactive thinking thinking ahead and anticipating events

procrastination putting things off until the last minute

profession an area of specialization

professional image enhancing and demonstrating one's professionalism; for example, by becoming actively involved in a professional organization

professionalism skills, traits, and other desired behaviors expected of someone trained to do a certain job

pronunciation the correctness with which words are pronounced

Protected Health Information (PHI) any health information, such as health status, payment, or patient status that can be linked to a specific individual

protocols guidelines and established ways of doing things within each health care organization

psychological abuse results in a fearful state for the person being abused; can be in the form of vicious threats

psychomotor domain one area of learning identified in Bloom's taxonomy. This domain focuses on performance of motor or hands-on activities, such as skills.

punctuality being on time

rapid eye movement (REM) a sleep stage in which the eyes move rapidly, characterized by dreaming

reactive thinking dealing with things after they occur

receiver the person for whom a message is intended

reframing changing the perception of a situation

respect valuing patients and coworkers by being courteous and understanding even in the most difficult situations

responsibility being accountable for your actions

résumé a short summary about oneself that informs potential employers about education, experience, and qualifications for the job

routes of transmission the various ways in which an infection can be spread

rumor information that has been presented as fact but has not been confirmed

sadness a state of sorrow and unhappiness

scope of practice written laws or statutes within each state that define what certified or licensed health care workers can do

selective comprehension focusing attention toward the part of a conversation that is most interesting during the communication process, while paying little attention to anything else

selective memory the process in which only certain things are remembered (usually the positive), while other things are forgotten

self-confident attitude focusing on the positive aspects of oneself to help accomplish goals in a positive manner

self-esteem personal feeling about oneself

self-motivation awareness of personal skills and abilities that are then developed to full potential; desire to achieve on your own

semantic barriers different meanings of a word or phrase between a sender and receiver that can cause misunderstanding of the message

sender the person delivering a message

service industry business providing a service to others

sexual abuse any inappropriate sexual touch or act

short-range goal a goal that can be achieved in the near future

sincerity honesty

social space the distance of 4 to 12 feet from a patient where initial rapport is established

standard precautions set of guidelines to prevent the spread of infection

STAT immediately

stress reaction an unpleasant emotional reaction to physical or psychological stress

synchronous distance education teacher and students interact in different places at the same time

tact consideration in interacting with others

telehealth the use of electronic communication between the provider and patient

telephone etiquette focusing attention on word choice and quality of voice during telephone conversations to ensure effective communication

territoriality the process of claiming certain space as one's own

time management skills set of skills to effectively organize tasks, prevent procrastination, and meet objectives on schedule

transmission-based precautions precautions specifically based on the route of transmission

trust consistent behavior that re-ensures the confidence of others, coworkers, and patients

trustworthy attitude the use of honesty, dependability, and responsibility to gain the trust of others

undirected thinking a free-flowing thinking process that can include both daydreaming and dreaming while asleep

upward communication initiated from the staff employees and flows upward to the person or persons in charge

values a person's beliefs, which are formed through thoughts, feelings, and actions

verbal abuse occurs when spoken words are meant to hurt another person's self-esteem

verbal communication the use of spoken words, as in conversations, oral reports, and voice mail, to communicate

vertical communication a combination of upward and downward communication

vertical thinking a logical type of thinking that makes step-by-step assumptions based on past experiences

victim attitude the continual attitude that "everything happens to me" and that one is helpless to change the situation

virtual learning also called e-learning, this is an electronic learning environment or platform

visualization to have a mental picture of something

web-based training training that occurs via the World Wide Web; can be synchronous, asynchronous, self-paced, instructor-led, or self-directed

worry to feel uneasy because of anxiety or troubles

written communication a form of communication that is written and organized in a precise and thorough manner; can include graphs, films, and reports

Index

Page numbers in *italics* refer to figures; and those followed by *t* indicate tables.